Faith and Fitness for Life

A 40-Day Transformational Journey

Lisa McCoy

A Not Forgotten Publication

Copyright © 2015 by Lisa McCoy

ISBN-13: 978-1-517-36113-6
ISBN-10: 1-517-36113-3

All rights reserved. No part of this book may be reproduced in any manner without written permission from the publisher, except in brief quotations used in articles or reviews.

Cover design by Lisa McCoy
Internal design and layout by Alice S. Morrow Rowan

Produced by
Not Forgotten Publishing Services
Not.Forgotten.Publishing@gmail.com

*For all of God's Daughters
who have ever struggled
with feeling valuable,
losing weight,
feeling healthy and strong,
knowing their Father's love,
living in freedom,
or claiming their identity
in Christ—*

this book is for you!

Contents

Acknowledgments vii
My Journey 1
Fasting and 40 Days 4
The 40-Day Plan 7
How to Get Started 14
The Covenant 17
Daily Devotions 19

- *Day 1*   What Did I Sign Up for? **21**
- *Day 2*   Desire **24**
- *Day 3*   Fight **27**
- *Day 4*   Give Me Food or Someone Is Going to Get Hurt! **30**
- *Day 5*   Good Health **33**
- *Day 6*   What Are You Afraid of? **37**
- *Day 7*   Friends in Losing Weight **41**
- *Day 8*   Adoption Day **44**
- *Day 9*   It's Not About the Gown, It's About the Crown! **47**
- *Day 10*   The Fat Kid **50**
- *Day 11*   Rose-Colored Glasses **54**
- *Day 12*   Who's Behind That Mask? **59**
- *Day 13*   The Real You **63**
- *Day 14*   Am I Beautiful? **66**
- *Day 15*   Addicted **71**
- *Day 16*   The Feeding Trough **75**

Day 17   Habit vs. Hunger   **80**
Day 18   Running for Comfort   **83**
Day 19   My Two Best Friends: Guilt and Shame   **87**
Day 20   Unraveling Anger   **91**
Day 21   Forgiveness Is NOT a Feeling   **95**
Day 22   Portion Distortion   **98**
Day 23   The Scale of Bondage   **102**
Day 24   Uncompromising in the Face of Temptation   **105**
Day 25   Planning for Profit   **109**
Day 26   Two Lies We Believe About Time and Priorities: Lie #1   **114**
Day 27   Two Lies We Believe About Time and Priorities: Lie #2   **119**
Day 28   Validated Through Approval   **123**
Day 29   Unwrapping Your Gift and Giving It Away   **127**
Day 30   Comparing Yourself to Others   **131**
Day 31   Give It a Rest!   **136**
Day 32   Listen When Your Body Is Speaking   **141**
Day 33   Dream Big   **145**
Day 34   W.A.I.T.   **150**
Day 35   Love Expressed   **155**
Day 36   Made in the Image of God   **160**
Day 37   Running Is Fun?   **165**
Day 38   Feed Your Faith, Not Just Your Face   **168**
Day 39   Pass It On!   **172**
Day 40   Time to Celebrate!   **176**

Glossary of Bible Translations   **180**

Acknowledgments

To my Lord and Savior Jesus Christ: I thank you for pushing me out of my comfort zone and transforming my life in ways I never imagined. To You be ALL the glory and honor!

To Tom, my husband: I could not have done this without your constant encouragement and comfort each step of the way. Thank you for believing in me and dreaming with me. Thank you for loving me in the midst of my struggles. But most of all thank you for stepping out of the boat with me!

To my family and friends: I thank you for your prayers, support, and understanding in the months of preparation for this book.

Faith and Fitness for Life

My Journey

Every journey has a beginning and an end. I like to think that my journey began in April 2014 when I did my first fast from the "white stuff." But honestly this journey began long before that. As far back as I can remember I was overweight and disappointed in how I looked. I never considered myself to be beautiful or attractive, and I felt very self-conscience about the shape of my body. My poor self-image led me into feeling worthless and to doubting that a man would ever love me, because who would love a fat girl?

For years I tried weight-loss programs, diet pills, and exercise systems with the hope of finally losing all the excess weight and becoming attractive. And I would lose weight on these programs, only to gain it back again plus more when I stopped the program. The roller-coaster ride of weight loss and gain also affected my emotions and dictated how I felt about myself. When I was losing weight I felt better about myself and was motivated to keep going, but as soon as my weight loss stopped or I gained weight or "cheated" on my diet, I would resign myself to the fact that I would never be thin, so I'd just give up. And when I gave up, my emotions spiraled into self-pity and depression, so I would eat to find comfort and hide the pain.

So what happened in March of 2014 to make me try again? Desperation! I was desperate for help and tired of being overweight and having no energy. I knew I couldn't do another weight-loss program just for the sake of losing pounds; I needed it to mean more so I wouldn't give up. So in my desperation I finally turned to the one source I knew would have the answer: God. I stopped pretending I was OK with my body weight and self-image, got real with God, and prayed for a solution to my situation. And what God revealed to me changed my life, my weight, my self-image, how I chose to eat, and best of all my relationship with my

Savior. You see, the problem wasn't any of those programs I had tried before; the problem was my heart.

Before, when I would set out on a journey to lose weight, my motivation was completely about me, how I wanted to look and how I saw myself, and the potential of gaining acceptance from others because I was thin. I relied on my own strength and willpower to sustain the program I was currently doing. I was proud of myself when I achieved success, and depressed when I fell short. My heart was totally focused on "self" and attaining the worldly goals of a perfect body image and perfect weight so I could feel good about the way I looked and finally be accepted as beautiful by others. But this time, in order for me to be successful I had to stop making my eating and exercise about me and make it about obedience to my Heavenly Father.

Scripture teaches us that as Christians our body is the temple in which the Holy Spirit lives. And we are to honor God and bring Him glory with our bodies, with what we eat and drink (1 Corinthians 6:19–20, 10:31) My heart was convicted in a way that I had never felt before. I wasn't bringing God glory with how and what I was eating, nor was I honoring Him with how I treated my body. What I was doing was trashing the temple. My heart's desire concerning food and how I looked was about what I wanted, not about what my Heavenly Father was asking of me or desired for me.

Beloved, I pray that in all respects you may prosper and be in good health, just as your soul prospers.
3 John 1:2 (NASB)

Our Heavenly Father wants good health and a prosperous soul for us. But I had to do my part. And my part was eating, exercising, and resting in a way that produced physical and spiritual health that would give me the strength and energy to live out my purpose and the call that God had placed on my life. My desire became what God had wanted for me all along: not to be defined by the world's standards of health and beauty but to become the woman He had designed me to be, defined by His Truth of health and beauty. Once I committed my eating to God, He began to reveal and then redeem my addiction to food and sugar, my poor eating habits, my distorted view of myself, and the lies I believed.

I can't say that my journey of faith and fitness is over or has been completed. But I can say that I am more equipped, healthier, stronger, and prepared. I can say that through the power of Jesus Christ I have been set free from the bondage that food had me in and from my addiction to sugar. He has renewed how I view my body and has captivated my heart with His great love. Every day I make the choice of what to eat, if I should exercise, and how I will spend time with Jesus. He has transformed my life by shedding the physical and spiritual pounds that were weighing me down and keeping me from being the person He had created me to be.

We can't do this without knowing why we are doing it. And what better reason is there than to honor and glorify our Heavenly Father? The blessings we receive are His promises of good health and a prosperous soul as we commit our eating, exercise, prayer, and rest to Him. I pray that you enjoy the days ahead and the good things you receive from the One who loves you the most: our Heavenly Father. ≈

Fasting and 40 Days

If you are like me, when you hear the word *fasting* the thought that follows is, "There's no way I can do that!" or "There's no way I can give that up!" And you would be right. We can't approach this time of fasting from certain foods by depending on our own strength. If we do, we are missing out on the potential blessings and breakthroughs that God wants to give us when we include Him in our fast. The concept of fasting, as seen in the Bible, is accompanied by prayer. The reason is that fasting was designed as a means of drawing closer and becoming more dependent on God, and prayer is one way of doing just that. "Draw near to God and He will draw near to you" (James 4:8, ESV).

When we fast and pray we are putting ourselves into the best possible place for a breakthrough. And that breakthrough, when it occurs, will be different for each of us. I was in desperate need of a breakthrough to lose weight so I could feel good about the way I looked. But the breakthrough that God had waiting for me was so much more. He wanted to break my addiction to food, reveal and redeem my emotional eating, and open the eyes of my heart to His Truth about how He had made me and how He sees me as beautiful. No matter what breakthrough you need, fasting and prayer have the potential to break the yoke of bondage and bring freedom to your soul (Isaiah 58:6). I believe that God wants to give you the blessing of a breakthrough that will forever change how you care for His temple, your body, and equip you with enough energy to fulfill His purpose in your life.

Fasting implies that we are giving up something in order to replace it with something else. For us that means giving up white sugar, white flour, white potatoes, white rice, corn, and artificial foods and replacing them with prayer and time in God's Word. In the following chapter, you will discover the research on and health benefits of removing these items from your diet.

After Jesus had fasted in the desert, He was tired, weak, and alone. And that is when the enemy showed up and began to tempt Him. In Jesus's physically weakened state, His only and most effective defense was speaking the Word of God. Knowing God's Truth gave Jesus the ability to resist temptation and defeat the enemy (Matthew 4:1–11). Make no mistake, Satan is very real and he will not want you to succeed. He will tempt you when you are most vulnerable, with the hope of blocking your breakthrough. Remember, temptation is not a sin until we give in to it and disobey God. So stand guard by staying focused on the scriptures provided in the devotional part of this book and on communicating with God through fervent prayer.

Why 40 Days?

In the Bible the number 40 is often associated with major changes and transformations, and it is always a period of testing, trial, and probation followed by restoration, revival, or renewal.

It rained 40 days and nights when God wanted to cleanse the earth and begin again (Genesis 7:12).

Moses spent 40 days on Mount Sinai on two separate occasions, once to receive instructions on building the tabernacle and once to receive the Ten Commandments (Exodus 24:18, Exodus 34:28–29).

The Israelites wandered in the wilderness for 40 years before entering the Promised Land (Exodus 16:35, Numbers 14:33–34).

For 40 days Goliath strutted in front of the Israelite army before being killed by David (1 Samuel 17:16).

Elijah, strengthened by one meal, traveled 40 days to Mount Horeb (1 Kings 19:8).

Jonah spent 40 days boldly warning the people of Nineveh that God would overthrow them if they did not turn from their evil ways (Jonah 3:4, 10).

Jesus fasted for 40 days in the wilderness before beginning His ministry (Matthew 3:17), and He appeared to His disciples for 40 days after His crucifixion and resurrection.

These are just some of the examples of the number 40 found in the Bible. In each example we see the transforming power of God and His ability to bring healing and renewal. And because we are seeking a transformation that will bring about a change in our lifestyle, we will follow the examples given to us by our Heavenly Father and fast and pray for 40 days, understanding that these 40 days will be a time of testing and trial so that we may find restoration, revival, and renewal for our physical and spiritual health. ≈

The 40-Day Plan

The 40-day plan of fasting and prayer consists of daily devotions, a list of foods and ingredients from which you will be fasting, exercise guidelines, and other tips to encourage your success.

Devotions and Prayer

In this book I have provided 40 devotionals, one for each day of your journey of prayer and fasting. I encourage you to start each day by reading the devotion and completing the Taking It to Heart section. These devotions and questions are meant to inspire you on your journey and to reveal those places that God wishes to redeem. I have also included daily prayers to guide you in your conversations with your Heavenly Father, and extra tips to help you in your commitment to caring for His temple, your body.

Accountability Partner or Group

> *Let us consider how we may spur one another on toward love and good deeds. Let us not give up meeting together, as some are in the habit of doing, but let us encourage one another—and all the more as you see the Day approaching.*
>
> Hebrews 10:24–25 (NIV)

God did not design you to walk your journey alone. We all need someone, or a group of people, who will offer us support, comfort us, encourage us, and speak the Truth in love to us during these 40 days. Prayerfully consider who can serve as your accountability partner or group. Even better, invite them to participate in the 40-day fast with you. Make the commitment to pray for each other daily, speak often during the week, take walks together a few days each week, or some combination of these.

40 Days of Fasting

For 40 days you will be fasting from white sugar, white flour, white rice, white potatoes, corn, and artificial foods. Each of these items is discussed in the following paragraphs to help you understand why you will take these particular items out of your diets for 40 days. I understand it may seem overwhelming to think about eliminating these foods from your diet, so instead of focusing on what you will be giving up, consider what you have the potential to gain. Your mind will be renewed by the daily mediation on scripture, your communication with God will be deepened through prayer, the abundant food that God has supplied for you will taste better than ever before, your energy will increase as your guilt over poor eating choices diminishes, and you will experience victory in those areas that God reveals and redeems.

White Sugar. In our house we refer to white sugar as "sweet poison." Although we laugh when we give that label to a food that contains refined sugar, there is truth to it. A poison is defined as something that has a harmful influence or that perverts. God has given us a natural form of sugar found in raw vegetables, raw fruits, honey, and maple syrup that provides nutrients to fuel the cells in our bodies. But we have perverted God's sugar by processing sugarcane and sugar beets to produce what we call refined sugar. During this refining process, all of the fiber, minerals, proteins, fats, and enzymes are removed, and all that is left are carbohydrates, or what we might call "empty calories," meaning there is no nutritional value in that caloric intake. So, according to the definition of poison, white sugar qualifies because it has been perverted away from its original state and the way God intended for us to enjoy it.

The other part of the definition of poison is that it has a harmful influence. So what is the harmful influence of sugar?

First, when we consume refined sugar our body must borrow vital nutrients, such as calcium, sodium, potassium, and magnesium, from various parts of our body to metabolize the sugar, thereby depleting the body's natural storage of these much-needed nutrients. And because 80 percent of the 600,000 food products we consume contain added refined sugar, according to the 2014 documentary *Fed Up*, our bodies are constantly being depleted of more and more of the nutrients needed to keep our health in balance. Due to this depletion, the body can't metabolize sugar, and poisonous waste accumulates in the brain, nervous system, and bloodstream, causing deterioration in our health. Our immune systems become suppressed and our risk of obesity, heart disease, and diabetes increases. Blood sugar levels spike and plummet, causing headaches, mood swings, and fatigue. Sugar can also cause tooth decay and gum disease, accelerate aging, and increase stress.

Second, sugar is addictive. Yes, you can be addicted to sugar. *Fed Up* shows a PET scan of a brain that consumes sugar, compares it to one that is addicted to cocaine, and points out that our brains "light up" from sugar just as they do from cocaine and heroin, thus causing addiction. Dr. David Rueben, author of *Everything You Wanted to Know About Nutrition*, writes that "white refined sugar is not a food. It is a pure chemical extracted from plant sources, purer in fact than cocaine, which it resembles in many ways." He goes on to share that for all practical purposes the chemical formula for cocaine differs from sugar in only one way, and that is that sugar does not have the nitrogen atom. We can actually get "high" on sugar. Consuming sugar can make us feel euphoric immediately, and if we don't get our sugar "fix," we can experience withdrawal symptoms, such as irritability, headaches, and other flu-like symptoms. We can become dependent on the effect that sugar has on us, thus becoming a sugar addict.

Removing sugar from your diet will be challenging at first. You may even experience symptoms of withdrawal. But hang in there: it will be worth it. What you gain will far outweigh what you give up.

White Flour. Here's another food fact for you: manufacturers take the beautiful whole wheat kernels that God has given us, strip away the health-giving fibers and nutrients—such as B-vitamins, bran, and wheat germ—and send what is left through a bleaching process to make what we call white flour. This final product is so nutritionally void that federal law requires the manufacturers to add certain vitamins back in, synthetically, and that's why we see the word *enriched* on our food labels. Because vitamins and fibers are missing from white flour products, the body will turn to its own tissues and bones to find the stored nutrients required for digestion of wheat. This body depletion can lead to blood sugar disorders that contribute to obesity, digestive issues, and inflammation that, depending on the individual, can result in arthritis, heart disease and other chronic diseases, memory loss, wrinkled skin, and diabetic complications.

Make sure you read your labels! Look for products made with whole grains; these will give you the fiber and nutrients needed to fuel a body that brings honor to your Heavenly Father.

White Rice, White Potatoes, and Corn. White rice, white potatoes, and corn all contain carbohydrates that quickly turn into sugar in our bodies, making us feel tired and potentially contributing to our being overweight. During these 40 days, as we try to break our food addictions and glorify God with our bodies, it is best to eliminate these "white foods" from our diets. Although carbohydrates are essential for good health and are fuel for our bodies, we should look for these in God-given carbs such as vegetables, fruits, legumes, and whole grains.

"Free" Foods and Artificial Ingredients. I'm sure that at one point or another we have all reached for food labeled fat-free or sugar-free in an attempt to eat healthier. But the truth is they are not free at all: our bodies pay the price for consuming these foods.

In sugar-free products, the sugar is replaced with artificial sweeteners that don't have any calories but are much sweeter than real sugar, and that confuses our bodies. When we eat something sweet our body expects calories to follow, but because the artificial sweeteners don't have any calories, our body goes looking for them later, which causes us to crave more and binge eat. The fat-free versions of the foods we enjoy simply replace the fat with sugar, and we have already learned about that "sweet poison."

Manufacturers also add flour, thickeners, and salt to enhance the flavor, but these in turn create more calories in our consumption.

Artificial sweeteners and flavors are just that: artificial. Studies have been done that show how they damage the body and negatively influence our mental health. Some of us have bought into the lie that artificial sweeteners are a good alternative to sugar, but the fact is, if we are honoring the temple, our body, and glorifying God in our diets, we need to stop eating food that our Heavenly Father did not make.

Stop Eating Three Hours Before Bedtime

Closing down the kitchen three hours before bedtime is one of the best actions you can take to promote good health and weight loss. Not eating during this period gives your body time to digest before going to sleep. Sleeping on a full stomach can make sleeping uncomfortable because the body is simultaneously shutting down to rest while still exerting energy to digest the food, leading to restlessness as well as gas and indigestion. Not eating before bed will also reduce your calorie intake, contributing to better weight management.

In the beginning of implementing this action you may find that you have low blood sugar headaches. Try drinking more water, or if you really need a snack, try a hard-boiled egg with a few slices of apple, or warm up a cup of low-sodium chicken or vegetable broth to drink.

Exercise Plan

You will be doing 20 to 30 minutes of moderate exercise five days a week.

> *For physical training is of some value, but godliness has value for all things, holding promise for both the present life and the life to come.*
>
> 1 Timothy 4:8 (NIV)

Notice that this verse doesn't say you don't need physical exercise. In fact, it tells you that physical exercise has value, but it prioritizes it by explaining that godliness has a greater value. Your focus in exercise should not be to improve your physical appearance so that others will notice and admire you; rather, the goal of exercise should be to improve your physical health so that you can gain strength and energy that can be devoted to your spiritual calling.

God designed your body to benefit from physical exercise. These are some of those benefits:

- More oxygen to the brain, which can heighten concentration and improve memory
- Reduced stress and anxiety levels
- Increased ability to fight depression
- More energy and strength
- Better sleep
- Enhanced immune system
- Lowered risk of heart disease, stroke, and diabetes
- Improved breathing
- Reduced body fat
- Slower aging process

Go ahead and treat yourself to moderate exercise, such as a walk, and enjoy the multiple benefits of your commitment to caring for God's temple, your body.

Hydrate

Your body needs a minimum of six to eight glasses of pure water per day. One of the best things you can do for yourself is to begin your day by drinking a glass of water on an empty stomach. I know it is not as appealing as that cup of coffee, but it will start your day right. While you have been asleep, your body has slowly been dehydrating because, well, you've been asleep and not drinking water. That morning glass of water will fire up your metabolism, hydrate you, and fuel your brain.

Beware of caffeinated drinks: they will dehydrate you. The average person consumes only one or two glasses of water a day, so you want to be sure to continue to hydrate with pure water throughout the day. Water helps to clean toxins out of your body, flushes fat, relieves water retention, gives you energy, creates beautiful skin, and even helps you to eat less. Proper water consumption is essential to your good health.

Get Proper Rest

According to the National Sleep Foundation, the average adult requires six to nine hours of sleep per night for good health. A good night's sleep is key to building a healthy lifestyle and can benefit your heart health, weight, and mind. But a good night's sleep is not the only form of rest. Your Heavenly Father has given you the command to keep a Sabbath. That means that during the week you need to take a break from your busy schedule and to-do list. I know it seems impossible to give up that time, but if you act in obedience to what your Heavenly Father has commanded and take a Sabbath, He will bless your obedience by restoring and multiplying your efforts the other days of the week. Proper rest is part of honoring God with your body, His temple. Make the commitment to get proper sleep each night, and take a Sabbath each week. ≈

How to Get Started

I am so excited that you have decided to listen to the call from your Heavenly Father and begin your journey to better health and a prosperous soul. Following is a checklist of how to prepare for 40 days of fasting and praying.

1. Read and sign The Covenant.

2. Consult a physician before starting the exercise and eating program.

3. Remember, you are fasting from

   - *White sugar and brown sugar.* Stevia, honey, pure maple syrup, and birch sugar, know as xylitol, are acceptable to use, but be careful not to overdo them. They are still forms of sugar and not meant to be consumed in large quantities.

   - *White flour and white flour products.* Brown rice flour and spelt flour are good substitutes. If you want to lose weight, try to stay away from yeast as well.

   - *White rice, white potatoes, and corn.* Instead use brown rice and brown rice pasta.

   - *"Free" foods and artificial sweeteners and ingredients.* Stay away from "fat-free" and "sugar-free" foods. Artificial sweeteners such as Splenda, NutraSweet, and any made with saccharin should be avoided. Try also to eliminate diet drinks and foods made with MSG and saturated fats.

4. Before beginning your fast, purge from your pantry and kitchen any food items that contain the foods from which you

How to Get Started

are fasting. I am not suggesting that you throw them away, but perhaps give them away or store them in a large container to keep them out of temptation's grasp. In order not to send your family into panic and shock over losing their favorite snacks and foods, consider placing your own food items in a cupboard set apart from the family's pantry during the 40 days of fasting and prayer—although I encourage you as wives and mothers to introduce the way you are eating to your family. Remember, you are aiming to transform your lifestyle, not just to diet, and what better gift can you give your loved ones than to show them the blessings and benefits of eating in a way that honors and glorifies God.

5. Take time each week to plan your meals and snacks before heading to the grocery store or farmer's market. This will help you to manage your time better and make grocery shopping and meal preparation easier. It will help you avoid unhealthy choices, eliminate stress over last-minute decisions about what to make for dinner, and save time, money, and calories. It will also enable you to enjoy variety, help you to avoid wasting food, and assist you in maintaining a healthy, balanced diet.

6. Pick one day a week to do your food preparation. It takes time to prepare food for healthy eating. Here a few tips to help you prepare for the weeks ahead.

- Cut up raw veggies and put them in storage bags or containers. Wash and dry lettuce, spinach, kale, and so on and store them in the refrigerator.

- Boil 2 to 4 chicken breasts, cool and dice them, and store them in the refrigerator or freezer for use during the week in salads and stir fries.

- Keep a bowl of apples on your kitchen counter for an easy snack.

- Make your own salad dressings or keep oil and vinegar on hand to dress your salads.

- Keep 6 to 8 hardboiled eggs on hand for an easy breakfast or quick protein snack or to use in a salad.

Other Encouraging Tips Before You Begin

- Try not to weigh yourself. Remember you are doing this for God's glory, not your own. Let honoring God be your motivation to continue, not the numbers on the scale.

- If you blow it on a meal or snack, don't condemn yourself or stress out over it. Go back and read the covenant you signed to remind yourself why you are fasting and praying, then get back on track and keep moving forward.

- The Faith and Fitness for Life Cookbook is a great resource for tasty recipes to get you started on your journey.

- You CAN do it! I believe that through the power and strength of Jesus Christ you can complete the 40 days of fasting and praying and experience freedom and victory like never before! ≈

The Covenant

A covenant is often thought to be a promise, but it is so much more than a promise. A promise is usually one-sided and dependant on only one of the parties doing something. It is also easily broken and doesn't mean there's a guarantee, like when my kids promise to clean their rooms but don't follow through.

A covenant, by contrast, is a binding agreement made between two parties and meant never to be broken. In the Bible, when a covenant was made between God and His people, the conditions were set by God with an expectation of certain conduct from them; man promised to keep those conditions and in return was blessed. For example, God's covenant with Noah was to never again destroy the earth by flood (Genesis 9:9–17); He promised Abraham that he would become the ancestor of a great nation if he went to the place that God showed him (Genesis 15); and God's covenant with Moses was that the Israelites would reach the Promised Land if they obeyed the Law (Exodus 24:4–8). In the New Testament, God promised salvation to those who believe in Jesus Christ (John 3:16, Romans 9:10).

God has given you the terms of how to care for your body, His temple, and He is expecting you to follow through on those terms. A written covenant with your Heavenly Father is a way of agreeing to those terms and committing your eating, exercise, and rest to honoring Him. Your diet and lifestyle become about His glory and not your own. And in Him you are blessed with the fruit of the Spirit and are becoming the person He created you to be.

Feel free to use the following covenant letter or write your own. I encourage you to sign it and hang it where you will see it every day as a reminder of your commitment to God and of His to you. ≈

The 40-Day Covenant

To my Heavenly Father,

I make a covenant with You to take care of Your temple, my body. I commit these 40 days to honoring You by fasting from all white sugar, white flour, white rice, white potatoes, corn, and artificial food. I also commit to giving up any other food or drink that is harmful to my body and does not bring You glory. I commit to eating healthy, balanced meals and snacks, to exercising in a way that honors Your temple, and to getting proper rest. I commit to daily prayer, to reading the devotional materials provided, and to completing the journaling. I do this all to bring You glory and not myself.

I know that by keeping my promise I can expect You to move and grow me in new ways, continuing to reveal the person You created me to be.

Beginning Date: _____

Ending Date: _____

Signed: _____

Witnessed and Supported by:

_____

Daily Devotions

Day 1
What Did I Sign Up for?

In March of 2014, while coming home with my husband from a family function, I began to sob uncontrollably. My precious husband, not knowing what to do with his hysterical wife, reached over, touched my knee, and with a deer-in-the-headlights look asked, "What's wrong?" Through my sobs and tears I told him how unhappy I was with how I looked and that I was tired of being overweight. My entire life was a battle with the bulge and I was done. I was giving up. I told my husband I couldn't do another weight-loss "program," fad diet, or crazy exercise plan. They didn't work for me. I needed something more. Whatever I did, I needed it to be about more than just losing weight so I could look good, because that seemed unattainable. It needed to mean something deeper than just following an exercise program and eating plan. I needed to be rescued from this crazy up-and-down cycle of weight loss and gain. I longed to be redeemed from my broken self-image. What I needed was a Savior.

So that's where I turned: to my Lord. And I actually started to get excited, not because of the promise of losing weight but because I had found my *why*,—the reason behind taking this journey. And for me that journey began right where you are now.

> *"Do you not know that your body is a temple of the Holy Spirit, who is in you, whom you have received from God? You are not your own, you were bought at a price. Therefore honor God with your body."*
>
> *1 Corinthians 6:19–20 (NIV)*

Why would Paul use the word *temple* to describe our bodies? He could have said *home* or *residence*. But he chose the word *temple*, because it is a sacred place, a place where God dwells. It is also where God is worshiped and honored. And because God lives there, it belongs to Him. God purchased our temple at the cross through His Son Jesus Christ. It was a steep price to pay.

Christ sacrificed His entire body and life for us through His death and resurrection, and now He is asking us to sacrifice those foods and habits that are not keeping His temple healthy. There is no sacrifice I could ever make that would be as great as the one Jesus made for me. The *why* for me was the realization that, as a daughter of the King, my body was created to be a temple for the Holy Spirit to live in and use to further the Kingdom of God, and how could He do that through a temple that had no energy and was often sick? I wanted to be stronger, healthier, and closer to God so that I could be physically and spiritually ready to fulfill the call He placed on my life.

Taking It to Heart

1. What is your *why?* What is your reason for taking this journey?

2. How would you describe the current state of your "temple"?

3. Finish this statement: By the end of this 40-day fast I will have....

Heavenly Father and Daughter Time

Pray that God will begin to restore your temple to be a place that will bring Him all the glory and honor.

Temple Tip for the Day

Remember, we are fasting from white sugar, white flour, white rice, white potato, corn, and any artificial foods. ≈

Day 2

Desire

Desire: a longing or a craving, as for something that brings satisfaction or enjoyment (www.dictionary.com)

I can honestly say that I find great satisfaction and enjoyment when I eat cake! Especially if it is chocolate cake or carrot cake or butter cake with raspberry filling or red velvet cake or—OK, basically any cake will satisfy my craving. And let me tell you, nothing—and I mean *nothing*—would stand between me and a piece of cake! Until this past year, when I discovered that I am gluten sensitive. Do you know what that meant? NO CAKE! Oh, the disappointment and despair!

But that did not stop me from quenching my craving for cake. I set out on a quest to find a gluten-free cake that would satisfy my longing. I researched and experimented with different flours and recipes. Some were tasty and some—well, let's just say, even the dog didn't care for them. But I kept going, determined to find a solution, focused on the goal of a perfect gluten-free cake that would taste like the "real thing."

I think it is safe to say that I was obsessed with cake. The problem with my cake desire/obsession was that it made me focus on my loss and on what I couldn't have, which left me feeling discouraged and in a pit of self-pity.

You may start to feel the same way—focused on the disappointment of what you've committed to fast from. You may have overwhelming cravings that seem to occupy your every thought. The solution? Matthew 6:21 says, "For where your treasure is, there your heart will be also" (NIV). What I didn't realize is that cake had become my treasure and that is where my heart was focused.

Day 2 ~ Desire

But cake could offer me nothing except a temporary fix. I needed to shift my focus.

Let us fix our eyes on Jesus, the author and perfecter of our faith, who for the joy set before him endured the cross, scorning its shame, and sat down at the right hand of the throne of God. Consider him who endured such opposition from sinful men, so that you will not grow weary and lose heart.

Hebrews 12:2–3 (NIV)

When we fix our eyes on Jesus, we are intentionally looking away from that which is distracting us and focusing on Him. In this time of fasting and praying, there will be distractions, things that will pull our focus away from the One who gives us strength and hope. These distractions can come in many forms; mine was focusing on what I couldn't have. And all distractions lead to the same place: weariness, loss of hope, and disappointment. But if you turn your eyes and heart to Jesus, by focusing on the promises found in His Word, and remember the opposition He endured and where He is now, you will find strength, hope, and joy.

Taking It to Heart

1. Looking back at your answers from Day 1, what distractions can you anticipate that could keep you from sticking to your *why* and achieving your goal for the 40 days?

2. What can you do to minimize those distractions?

Heavenly Father and Daughter Time

Sit quietly today with your Heavenly Father, fix your eyes and mind on Him, and allow His presence to strengthen and refresh you.

Temple Tip for the Day

Focus on the bounty of beautiful, natural food that God has created for us. ≈

Day 3

Fight

My stepson is a U.S. Marine. Ooh-rah! We are so proud of his choice and commitment to serve and defend our country. He spent 13 weeks at the Parris Island, South Carolina, boot camp to earn the title of U.S. Marine. The boot camp consisted of intense, fierce physical and mental conditioning and training 24 hours a day, 7 days a week. The recruits' bodies were pushed to the limits to build endurance. They were trained in how to use weapons properly. Their minds were conditioned to follow orders without question, and they were disciplined when they didn't do something correctly or up to Marine standards. Even now as a U.S. Marine he continues his training and conditioning. Why? To prepare for battle—a battle that may or may not come. Either way, he is prepared.

His experience makes me think about how we prepare ourselves for battle. And make no mistake: we have an enemy and he is waging war on us. He does not want our bodies and minds in battle-ready condition. "Your enemy prowls around like a roaring lion looking for someone to devour" (NIV), Peter 5:8 says. I don't know about you but to me a roaring lion is an intimidating enemy. The only lion I've ever seen has been in a cage at the zoo, but I tell you this: if I saw one prowling around outside my house, you would find me inside behind locked doors dialing 9-1-1!

Peter warns us that this is exactly what the enemy is doing: prowling, searching for prey to ravenously swallow up. His roar, which is not always loud but is definitely heard above all else, is the lies we believe about our appearance, our emotions, and our diets, and he fills our ears with words of doubt, challenging us to believe we can't do this. The enemy does all of this to tempt us to unlock the door to our heart and let him in. And as soon as we unlock that door by believing a lie and giving up—BAM! We are devoured.

But we are not defenseless against this attack. As daughters of the King we are given access to the full armor of God. A belt of truth, a breastplate of righteousness, feet ready to move with the Gospel, a shield of faith, a helmet of salvation, and the sword of the Spirit, which is the Word of God. But having access doesn't mean we have put on that armor or used it. Ephesians 6:11 tells us to *"put on* God's whole armor [the armor of a heavily armed soldier that God supplies], that you may be able successfully to stand up against [all of] the strategies *and* the deceits of the devil" (AMP).

So how do we prepare for battle against the strategies and deceits of the devil? Like my stepson the U.S. Marine, we train! We grab the whole armor of God that He has supplied, put it on, and learn how to use it. We study His Word and continually communicate with our Father to nourish and strengthen our souls. We exercise and eat whole foods to nourish and strengthen our bodies. We do all of this in order to be fit to fight the enemy, so that when those battles come we can stand firm and fight in the strength and power of the Holy Spirit.

Taking It to Heart

1. Yesterday you listed those things that might potentially distract you from moving forward toward your goals. How might the enemy use those distractions to attack your efforts?

2. What spiritual weapon will you use to prepare for those attacks? And how will you use it? (Refer to Ephesians 6:14–18.)

Heavenly Father and Daughter Time

Each morning, put on the armor of God by praying Ephesians 6:14–18.

Temple Tip for the Day

Make sure to do 20 to 30 minutes of moderate exercise 5 days a week. ≈

Day 4

Give Me Food or Someone Is Going to Get Hurt!

I remember it was a Wednesday the first time I started this fasting and praying. The turmoil I felt inside drove me crazy. My emotions went from irritability to wanting to cry. I was overly sensitive and overreactive. Images would flash through my mind of little devil creatures pulling and clawing at me and hurling accusations that I would never lose weight and I wouldn't be able to stick with the plan. And then I would get these cravings and feel like I could rip open everything in the pantry and devour everything in the kitchen. I thought I was going insane.

But I wasn't going crazy; I was experiencing symptoms of withdrawal. When you remove white sugar, white flour, white rice, white potatoes, corn, and artificial foods from your diet, you may experience withdrawal symptoms such as anxiety, irritability, headaches, cravings, depression, and flu-like symptoms, just to name a few. But withdrawal wasn't the only trouble I was facing. I was becoming increasingly aware that the enemy had a strong grip on my mental and emotional attitude toward food, and he was not going to let go so easily.

The "crazy" state I was in that day was overwhelming to me. In those moments I would try to turn to God and pray or utter His name, and that seemed to help. But the moments were many and the fight, which I knew had just begun, was making me weary.

In John 16:33, Jesus is speaking to His disciples: "I have told you these things, so that in me you may have peace. In this world you will have trouble. But take heart! I have overcome the world" (NIV).

Day 4 ~ Give Me Food or....

Jesus has overcome the world! He hasn't promised that life with Him will be without challenges; in fact, He tells us we will have trouble. But He also tells us to have courage because the One who has defeated our enemy and claimed victory over every battle is the One who stands with us when trouble hits.

That day I knew the Lord was right there with me, and when I turned to Him in prayer He whispered these beautiful words to me, and I hope they will speak to your heart in the midst of your troubles, whether you are experiencing withdrawal or an attack of the enemy. He said to me, "Fear not, my child; I have overcome this already for you. Lean on me, stand behind me, hide in me, and I will tear down the enemies that are keeping you from fully experiencing the freedom that is found only in Me."

Taking It to Heart

1. What "trouble" are you facing today?

2. Can you recognize the true Victor in your trouble even though you may not "feel" victorious just yet?

3. How will you find courage and peace in the midst of trouble?

Heavenly Father and Daughter Time

Seek God's Word today and find a scripture that you can pray when faced with temptation, withdrawal, and attacks of the enemy. Write that scripture on a card and place it where you can see it or carry it with you.

Temple Tip for the Day

Withdrawal symptoms vary in time and experience. You may have headaches, anxiety, irritability, cravings, depression, dizziness, and flu-like symptoms, to name a few. To help resolve those symptoms, drink more water, drink more water, and drink more water! ≈

Day 5

Good Health

> *Beloved, I pray that in all respects you may prosper and be in good health, just as your soul prospers.*
>
> 3 John 1:2 (NASB)

John, one of Jesus's disciples, wrote this to his dear friend Gaius. Gaius was known for his hospitality and generosity toward traveling teachers and missionaries. It is thought that during John's travels Gaius had shared his home and hospitality with him. If so, John would have been grateful and would have written this personal letter of encouragement to Gaius. John wanted to encourage both his spiritual and his physical health. When this letter was written, popular opinion taught the separation of the spiritual and the physical. Today we still often hold this view, that there is *not* a connection between the physical and spiritual sides of our being. This attitude can likely lead to neglect of the body, of the spirit, or of both, or to overindulgence of the body's sinful desires.

My actions throughout my life would fall into both of these categories. First, there is the side of me that would overindulge. I have done this in many ways over the years. I would overindulge by eating whatever I wanted and however much I wanted, or I would be obsessed with insane workouts to lose weight. But then I would also neglect taking care of my body by making excuses that sounded very spiritual, like "This must just be how God wants me to be" or "This obviously is how God made me and I should learn to accept who I am at whatever weight I am" or "It's what's on the inside that's more important." Granted, parts of these statements are true: God did design me to be me and, yes, I should accept that God has made me fearfully and wonderfully in

His image and, yes, the condition of my heart, the inside, is important. But in all honesty I was never thinking of God's Truth when I spoke those words or chose to overindulge. What I was doing was giving up and giving in! I was giving up on ever losing weight and ever having peace about how I look. I was giving in to what I desired at any given time. Neither giving up nor giving in has anything to do with God's Truth and what He desires for me—and for you.

What God desires for us are good health and a soul that is prospering. So what does God mean by "good health" and a "prospering soul"? "Good health" refers to the physical state of our bodies. It is not the absence of disease or sickness but rather a body strengthened by daily physical exercise, good nutrition, and adequate rest. Our souls are the seat of our emotions, so a prosperous soul is one that has well-balanced emotions that help you to thrive. God is concerned with both our body and our soul. He has connected them on purpose for a purpose. Our soul is where God ignites our passions and dreams, and our body is the vehicle that carries out those passions and dreams in the service of our King. So, by caring for your physical needs, disciplining your body, and nurturing your soul, you will be able to be at your best for God's service.

Taking It to Heart

1. On a scale of 1 to 7, with 7 being the best and 1 being the worst, how would you rate your physical health (eating and exercise)?

2. How have you overindulged or neglected your physical health?

3. What reason or excuse have you used to overindulge or neglect your physical health?

4. On a scale of 1 to 7, with 7 being the best and 1 being the worst, how would you rate your soul's health (devotions, prayer, etc.)?

5. How have you overindulged or neglected your soul's health?

6. What reason or excuse have you used to overindulge or neglect your soul's health?

Heavenly Father and Daughter Time

Take your reasons and excuses for overindulging and/or neglecting to your Heavenly Father. Lay them at the foot of the cross and ask Him to replace your excuses and reasons with His truth and His purpose.

Temple Tip of the Day

Write this scripture on a card and place it where you will see it each day. Read it as a reminder of God's desire for you:

> [*Your name*], *I pray that in all respects you may prosper and be in good health, just as your soul prospers.*
> 3 John 1:2 (NASB) ≈

Day 6
What Are You Afraid of?

When I was a little girl we lived in an old farmhouse. I loved my bedroom in that old house—except for one feature: the door to the attic. It was a fullsize door in the far corner of the room, and my bed was positioned directly across from it, in full view of it. For some reason I feared that attic door, or I should say, I was afraid of what *might* be behind it. Interestingly, I was afraid of that attic door only at nighttime. As I would lie in my bed trying to fall asleep, my imagination would come up with some pretty shady characters that might be living in our attic. There might be ghosts or maybe even aliens living in our attic—or worse, maybe the bogeyman! I was so afraid that in order to fall asleep I would pull the blanket up over my head, convinced that if these shady characters were to escape from the attic and into my room, they wouldn't see me.

And then one night my worst fear was confirmed. A windy, thunder-and-lightning storm was brewing as I got into bed. Our old farmhouse would creak and bend when it was windy. So there I lay, tucked into bed, lightning flashing and the wind howling, blanket pulled up to my nose, with only my eyes showing. Then suddenly the attic door flew open, and in a fear-driven panic I dove under the covers. At that point I could only imagine what was coming out of the attic: a ghost, an alien, the bogeyman. I will never know what, or if anything at all, came out of the attic that night, because I stayed hidden under the blanket, with my eyes tightly closed, paralyzed with fear, until morning.

Now, as an adult recalling that memory of my childhood, I laugh, thinking how silly I was to be so afraid of the attic and what *might* be lurking there. But then I realize that even as an adult fear can still paralyze me. I can still convince myself that what *might* lie

Faith and Fitness for Life

ahead is overwhelming and impossible. I can focus on the pressure of the situation, and I can allow my thoughts to drift into self-doubt. When I first set out on the journey of fasting and prayer to change to a healthy lifestyle, I was afraid. I was afraid that once again I would fail to lose any weight, afraid that I couldn't stick to the plan, afraid that I would disappoint God. But there is a remedy for our fear.

> *David also said to Solomon his son, "Be strong and courageous, and do the work. Do not be afraid or discouraged, for the Lord God, my God, is with you. He will not fail you or forsake you until all the work for the service of the temple of the Lord is finished."*
>
> *1 Chronicles 28:20 (NIV)*

Don't focus on the fear, and take a step forward! This is a remedy to our fears. It is so easy to allow our fears to consume our thoughts to the point where we become immobilized. It is so easy to focus on the possibilities of failure or on our perceived inabilities when faced with a new task. But that is why David reminds us that God will not fail us; God is with us as we complete the task ahead of us to which He has called us. We can find strength and courage when we take our eyes off of our fear and place them on God. But God also tells us to "do the work." Take that next step forward. But taking that next step will require trust in God, believing that what He says is true, that He will not fail us and is right there with us. And through our trust in God and our belief in His promises, we will find courage to move forward in the direction He is asking us to go.

Taking It to Heart

1. What fear are you facing right now that could stop you from moving forward on this journey?

2. What is the source of that fear?

3. How have you overcome fear before in your life?

4. What can you take from that previous experience in overcoming fear and apply to now?

5. What is the one "next step" that you can take to alleviate that fear?

6. When will you take that next step?

Heavenly Father and Daughter Time

Take your fear to your Heavenly Father, thank Him for never leaving you, and praise Him for never failing you.

Temple Tip of the Day

Exchange your dinner plate for a salad plate on which to eat your meals. And don't go back for seconds. ≈

Day 7
Friends in Losing Weight!

Congratulations! You've made it one week! I hope you take a moment and celebrate this milestone.

I had been maintaining a new lifestyle of healthy eating and exercise for 10 months when a group of ladies from my church asked if I would organize a group and walk with them as we fasted from the "white stuff" and prayed and exercised. I agreed and was happy to do this for them and with them, but what I didn't expect was the lesson I would learn from them. From this beautiful group of women I learned the value of being in a community of Believers.

We held each other accountable, became cheerleaders when we grew frustrated or weary, and grew stronger because we believed in each other. We prayed for each other, cried with each other, and celebrated every victory in Jesus's name! I learned that I am not alone in my struggle with food, weight loss, and self-image.

> *Therefore, since we are surrounded by such a huge crowd of witnesses to the life of faith, let us strip off every weight that slows us down, especially the sin that so easily trips us up. And let us run with endurance the race God has set before us.*
>
> Hebrews 12:1 (NLT)

My "crowd of witnesses" was this group of God's daughters who brought their life experiences and attitudes of encouragement together to create a safe place to lose weight. For some of us, the weight we wanted to lose was in pounds; for others it was an addiction to food, or poor eating habits, or a necessary adjustment due to physical illness. No matter what kind of "weight loss" we each faced, the common denominator was that the weight was slowing us down in the particular race God had designed for each of our lives. That weight can be physical or spiritual or both, and according to Hebrews 12:1, living the Christian life requires giving up whatever is endangering or interfering with our relationship with God. This is why God encourages us to be in community with other Believers—so that in our challenges we have others whom we can lean on and learn from, and so that we can do the same for them.

Taking It to Heart

1. Who is in your "crowd of witnesses"? Those who support you, encourage you, and pray for you.

2. How are you benefiting from being in a community of Believers?

3. What contributions do you bring to your community group?

Heavenly Father and Daughter Time

Take time to pray for each member of your "crowd of witnesses." Praise God for their love and friendship. Thank God for how they are speaking into your life.

Temple Tip of the Day

Take time this week to connect with one member of your "crowd of witnesses," thank them, pray with them, and even take a walk with them. ≈

Day 8

Adoption Day

Do you know that you were adopted? That used to be the question I would ask my little brother when we were kids. He is six years younger than I am, and until he came along I was an only child. And I liked it that way. I had all the love and attention of my parents. But when he was born, all of a sudden I had to share that love and attention with him. I did not think that was fair. I was here first. Shortly after he was born I requested that we send him back. My parents ignored my request with laughter, thinking it was just a phase and an adjustment time in my life. That phase was not a short one and I was not adjusting. So I changed my tactics. When he got a little older I would tell him that he was adopted. I didn't say it to make him feel loved and special; I said it to freak him out in the hope that he would run away and find his "real" family. My plan did not work. He stayed, and now I am so thankful that he did. Even though it wasn't my choice to have him join our family and at first it seemed like a curse, I learned that there was enough love and attention for both of us and that it was God's desire that he be a part of our family, just like it was God's desire that I too was a part of our family.

So I ask again, did you know that *you* are adopted?

For you are all children of God through faith in Christ Jesus.

Galatians 3:26 (NLT)

When we place our faith in Christ Jesus and accept Him as our Lord and Savior, we are instantly adopted by God into His family. And through that Heavenly adoption we become a daughter of the

Day 8 ~ Adoption Day

King. But our adoption was not free; a price was paid for it—a loving, lavish price.

> *See what great love the Father has lavished on us, that we should be called children of God! And that is what we are!*
>
> *1 John 3:1 (NIV)*

Our Heavenly Father's own Son paid the price for our adoption with His death on the cross and His resurrection from the grave. He showed a love without limits, a lavish love, and a great love given so that you and I can be called daughters of God.

Taking It to Heart

1. How does it feel to know that the price paid for your adoption into the family of God was the loving sacrifice of Jesus's life?

2. How can that feeling motivate you in this time of fasting?

Heavenly Father and Daughter Time

Take time today to recall the moment you placed your faith in Christ Jesus and accepted Him as your Lord and Savior. Celebrate that moment with an offering of praise to your Heavenly Father.

If you have not placed your faith in Christ Jesus and would like to do so, offer this heartfelt prayer as a repentance for your sin and as acceptance of Jesus as your Lord and Savior:

> *Lord Jesus, I know that I am a sinner. I believe in my heart that You died for my sins and rose from the grave so that I could have eternal life. I ask that you forgive me for my sins. Starting today I trust and follow You as Lord and Savior of my life. Thank you, Lord, for saving me and forgiving me. In Jesus's name I pray. Amen.*

If this was the first time you prayed this prayer, please contact a local pastor or your accountability partner to share in the celebration of this moment and get connected with the family of God.

Temple Tip of the Day

Eat more water-rich foods such as tomatoes, melons, and celery, which can help to fill you up without adding too many calories.

Day 9

It's Not About the Gown, It's About the Crown!

I have a friend who just could not picture herself as a princess. She couldn't shake the vision of the Disney version of what a princess looks like: sparkling skin, flawless figure, gorgeous hair, and a beautiful, flowing gown, not to mention the tiara. She just could not imagine herself in that way. Well, my goodness, who in real life could other than my 7-year-old niece? Like so many little girls, my beautiful niece has an active fantasy world where she believes she is a princess acting out her royal duties, which to her would be twirling in her ball gown, riding in make-believe carriages, and sipping tea. And if you watch my niece as she takes on her princess persona, it is not just the outside stuff that makes her feel like a princess. When she begins to act out her fantasy, you can see her demeanor change. She stands taller, becomes more graceful and gentle, and has confidence in who she is.

But somewhere between the ages of 7 and 40-something, our fantasy of being a princess is dismissed as merely that—a fantasy. Our skin doesn't seem to sparkle, we see our figures as flawed, and we have bad-hair days. Maybe once or twice we dress up in a pretty dress for a prom or a wedding. But being a princess is not defined by the gown; it's defined by the crown.

A crown is a symbol of identity, a symbol of who we truly are. As daughters of the King, God's princesses, our crowns symbolize our identity in Him; they stand for eternal life and show that we belong to Him.

Faith and Fitness for Life

Everyone who competes in the games goes into strict training. They do it to get a crown that will not last, but we do it to get a crown that will last forever.

1 Corinthians 9:25 (NIV)

Our journey of fasting, exercise, and prayer is how we are currently competing in the game of life. It is our "strict training." It is not training that brings us satisfaction in how much we weigh or in how we look. We aren't training so that we may gain man's approval or awards, for all those things fade away. It is training that equips us for life and prepares our hearts so that we may wear the crown bestowed on us by our Heavenly Father in a way that says, "I belong to God and to Him be all the glory."

Taking It to Heart

1. Describe how it makes you feel to know that you are God's princess.

2. What does it mean to you to wear an eternal crown that was given to you by your Heavenly Father?

3. How will this knowledge motivate you in moving forward in this time of fasting, exercise, and prayer?

Heavenly Father and Daughter Time

Spend time praising your Heavenly Father for crowning you as His own princess, His daughter. Pray that He begins to reveal your identity in Him and prepare your heart to live a life that glorifies the Father.

Temple Tip for the Day

Muscle burns more calories than fat, and strengthening muscle can increase your metabolism. Try to add 20 minutes of strength training to your exercise routine two to three times a week. ≈

Day 10

The Fat Kid

That's who I was: the fat kid. From Kindergarten through High School, that was the label I wore—*fat kid*. It was not a label I wore with pride. It was a label that crushed my spirit and made me feel ugly and unwanted. It was a label I carried into my adult life and allowed to shape my thinking about who I am.

By the time I hit my mid-20s, I fully believed that I was physically unattractive and no man would ever desire or love me. When I looked at myself I saw nothing beautiful. I saw only a fat girl whom no one would ever want. I felt lonely, unworthy, and unloved.

When I look back through my life's journey, I wonder where that label came from. Sure, a few kids throughout my childhood would tease me and call me names, but were those few encounters enough to influence my perception of myself? Those cruel words from a few individuals did wound my heart, but most wounds heal, unless they become infected. And that's what happened. My "fat kid" wound became infected—infected with lies.

Author Ron Keck has developed this model of how our hearts are captured and then enslaved to a lie: Strategic *arrows* are launched into our lives to create wounds–arrows like a difficult loss, painful circumstance, traumatic event, abuse, and so on. Our wounds become infected with *lies,* or false beliefs. Satan repeats the lies until we make *agreements* and accept them as truth. Once agreements are made, *vows* soon follow. The false agreements and vows feed the false self, and our views about ourselves become distorted and the masks we wear to cover our true selves.

My arrow was the label "fat kid" that created the wound in which Satan could whisper lies such as "No one loves a fat person,"

Day 10 ~ The Fat Kid

"You are ugly," "There's nothing special about you," "Because you are fat, you are worthless," just to name a few that I heard over the years. I started to believe those lies and agreed with them, then vowed that I would never let myself fall in love because the person I loved would never love me back and from now on I would be single and safe. Those lies I agreed with and the vow I made gave me a false view of myself—fat, ugly, unlovable, undesirable, worthless, and alone—and I hid my broken heart in food and pretended I felt good about who I was and how I looked while trying to keep my hurt hidden from everyone and myself.

So, how do we heal a wound that has been infected with lies? We learn what the Truth is and replace those lies with the Truth.

Jesus said . . . "If you continue in My Word, you really are my disciples. You will know the Truth and the Truth will set you free."

John 8:31–32 (HCSB)

When we spend time in God's Word, we learn the Truth of who we are in Christ and are equipped to recognize and rebuke the lies that have trapped us in false beliefs about ourselves. And when we know and accept the Truth, we are freed from the lies and can begin to allow Christ to heal our wounds.

The healing of spiritual wounds, like physical wounds, takes time and requires purposeful action on our part. When we have a cut in our flesh, we don't apply a healing ointment just once. We repeatedly apply the ointment until the cut is healed. So, in order for the wounds in our hearts, created from our false labels, to be healed, we have to keep applying the healing salve of God's Truth to them. We must continually write His Truth on our hearts so that we don't fall back into believing the lie. When we have a thought or hear a comment that is an attempt to reopen that wound, we can turn to Jesus and His Truth and keep reading it, saying it, and praying it until it becomes louder and stronger than the lie. That is how the Truth will set us free!

Taking It to Heart

1. What false labels are you carrying that have wounded your heart?

2. What lies have infected your wound that you are in agreement with?

3. What vows have you made?

Day 10 ~ The Fat Kid

4. How have those agreements and vows distorted your view of yourself?

5. How would you feel if you were free from that false belief about yourself?

Heavenly Father and Daughter Time

Seek God's Truth that speaks against the false labels that have wounded your heart. Write those scriptures on a card or paper and read them every day until that Truth is louder and stronger than the lies! Challenge yourself to memorize a scripture so that you can recall it in your time of need.

Temple Tip of the Day

A three-digit number does not have to be your weight-loss goal. Instead, let your goal be a dress size or waist measurement. ≈

Day 11

Rose-Colored Glasses

Have you ever heard a common phrase and wondered where it came from or what it really means? OK, maybe it's just me who does that. In any case, one day I decided to look up what the phrase *rose-colored glasses* actually means and where it came from. I was pleasantly reassured that how I had been using the phrase was correct; at the same time, I was amazed at the possibilities of how it originated. No one knows for sure where this phrase came from, but one explanation is this: because mapmakers of the 17th century had to pay close attention to detail, they would use rose petals to clean their lenses, and the rose petals would leave behind natural oils that would protect and stain the lenses. In this context, viewing the world through rose-colored glasses means focusing on the smaller details while ignoring the bigger view. Another explanation is that by the 19th century people were deliberately wearing tinted lenses in order to alter their view of reality, giving us the concept of choosing to see the world through optimistic eyes and ignore the negative circumstances around us. A much more bizarre explanation is that rose-colored goggles were designed for chickens to wear to prevent them from seeing blood on other chickens, in an attempt to decrease their aggressive behavior toward injured chickens.

I admit that last one is a little out there, but in all of the explanations the common thread is that looking through rose-colored glasses alters our perception, allows us to choose to focus on one particular aspect of our environment while ignoring the bigger picture and giving us an overly optimistic view of the world around us. Being optimistic is not a bad thing, but when our optimism is a way to deliberately ignore the negative or not-so-

Day 11 ~ Rose-Colored Glasses

pleasant aspects of our world, ourselves, or our circumstances, it becomes a form of denial or delusion and prohibits us from seeing the bigger, real picture.

I loved my rose-colored glasses. In fact, I loved them so much I wore them all the time, because they allowed me to see the attributes of myself that I liked and ignore those that I found disappointing. I was able to focus on my eyes and hair—my favorite parts—and ignore the rest of my body, which I didn't want to look at because it made me feel bad about myself. I was able to focus on my spiritual journey and ministry and ignore my poor self-image. The problem with looking at ourselves through rose-colored glasses is that we are seeing ourselves through the lenses of our past hurts, betrayals, experiences, and negative nurturing. We are not seeing our true selves, the way our King sees us.

"Your eye is a lamp that provides light for your body. When your eye is good, your whole body is filled with light. But when your eye is bad, your whole body is filled with darkness."

Matthew 6:22–23 (NLT)

If your eyes are open and you can see clearly, your body will be full of light. Look around you: you will see light! If you close your eyes, you will see darkness. Jesus uses this basic principle to show us that the eye is the center of our perception. Our eye is not the light itself but it is how light enters our bodies and guides our motions. But Jesus is speaking not just about our physical eyes. He is also speaking about our spiritual eyes, the pathway by which God's light enters and allows us to see and understand spiritual Truth. Once we see and understand His Truth, we can clearly see His vision and direction.

Now, we know that when we are seeing clearly our vision is focused. If our vision is not focused, what we see is blurry. When Jesus says, "when your eye is good," He is speaking about the focus of our vision. A focused vision is singular in nature, meaning it has a singleness of devotion, attention, and heart.

When we choose to view ourselves through rose-colored glasses, our spiritual vision becomes blurred—blurred by our unhealed hurts, the false labels we believe about ourselves, our unmet expectations of how we should look, and our negative experiences. Our blurred vision hinders God's Light, Jesus, from entering our body and filling us with the light of spiritual understanding of how God views us. And without that light we are in the dark, a place of delusion and denial.

Wearing our rose-colored glasses is an attempt to deny how we truly see and feel about ourselves. It is how we use our optimism to hide our hurt. It is how our "good eye" gets out of focus and can't see God's Truth about how He views us.

Open my eyes to see wonderful things in Your Word.

Psalm 119:18 (TLB)

Just as we see the light around us and it guides our body's movement, our spiritual eyes need the one true Light, Jesus, to guide the movement of our mind and heart. In both cases, the physical and spiritual, we must *choose* to take off our rose-colored glasses and open our eyes to let in the light, God's Truth. If we choose to keep them closed, we are in darkness and there is no light in us. And when we stand in darkness we cannot see who we truly are.

Taking It to Heart

1. How have you been wearing rose-colored glasses when looking at your physical self and spiritual self?

Day 11 ~ Rose-Colored Glasses

2. How has that view blocked you from seeing the "real" you?

3. Why do you choose to look at yourself through rose-colored glass?

4. What do you believe God sees when He looks at you, His Daughter?

5. What would it feel like to see yourself as God sees you?

6. What step(s) can you take to remove your rose-colored glasses and see yourself through God's Truth, the way He sees you?

Heavenly Father and Daughter Time

First choose to take off your rose-colored glasses and open your eyes. Then pray that the light of your Heavenly Father will fill you with all Truth.

Temple Tip for the Day

Don't skip meals. It will cause your body to go into starvation mode, making it hard to burn calories. Try eating 3 healthy meals a day and 2 to 3 healthy snacks. ≈

Day 12

Who's Behind That Mask?

Wonder Woman: she was my all-time favorite superhero growing up. She could spin around and transform herself from Diana Prince into Wonder Woman. She was beautiful and armed with a magic belt that gave her super strength, wristbands that could deflect bullets, an unbreakable lasso that could make anyone tell the truth, and a tiara that could be thrown as a weapon and then return to her like a boomerang. She was awesome!

But there was also something peculiar about Diana Prince and her superhero persona: no one recognized her as Diana when she was Wonder Woman, and vice versa. This puzzled me because the only difference between the two was the wardrobe. And she didn't wear a mask, yet no one recognized her as being the same person. It was almost as if she was wearing an invisible mask that could hide her identity.

Of course it seems impossible, except in the comics and on TV, that someone could walk around and not be seen for the person she really is. Yet how many of us wear an invisible mask that hides our true feelings, thoughts, and identity? If Wonder Woman's secret identity had been revealed, it would have made her vulnerable to her enemies. Perhaps that is why we hide our feelings, thoughts, and identity: to protect ourselves. For if our true feelings, thoughts, and identity were revealed, we would become vulnerable, and being vulnerable means we might get hurt. And no wants to get hurt.

But God sees us. He sees the deepest parts of us. No mask we try to wear can hide our true feelings and thoughts from Him. He longs for us to understand that He sees and hears our best and worst and will never reject or hurt us. In fact, He wants us to be vulnerable—vulnerable to His love and comfort.

> *O Lord, you have examined my heart and know everything about me. You know when I sit or stand. When far away you know my every thought. You chart the path ahead of me and tell me where to stop and rest. Every moment you know where I am. You know what I am going to say before I even say it. You both precede and follow me and place your hand of blessing on my head. This is too glorious, too wonderful to believe! I can never be lost to your Spirit! I can never get away from my God!*
>
> Psalm 139:1–7 (TLB)

God knows our secret thoughts and feelings about how we look, what we weigh, and what we eat. God knew I hated the way I looked. He saw my addictive eating habits. He heard my thoughts of disappointment and disgust every time I saw my body in the mirror or in a picture. He saw right through my mask into my pain and said, "I will never leave you or forsake you. I will guide you through this and my strength will support you every step of the way." So I trusted in His Word and took off my mask. I stopped trying to hide my true feelings and thoughts from the One who could heal them. And when I stopped hiding behind my mask, I became vulnerable to His love, comfort, and Truth. And that is when I began to see and accept the person God made as me.

Taking It to Heart

1. What feeling or thought about yourself are you hiding behind your mask?

Day 12 ~ Who's Behind That Mask?

2. Why do you want to hide that feeling or thought?

3. How would it feel to remove that mask and let God's Truth comfort you and heal you?

4. What is stopping you from removing that mask?

5. What can you do to minimize that roadblock to taking off your mask?

6. How does it feel to know that God knows your most secret thoughts and feelings about yourself and still loves you?

Heavenly Father and Daughter Time

Take off your mask and share your hurt and pain with your Heavenly Father. Ask Him to begin healing your hurt. Know that He is with you through every step.

Temple Tip for the Day

Store-bought salad dressings can be packed with calories and artificial foods. Make your own vinaigrette and keep it in a spray bottle to coat your salad with to avoid overdressing it, or use the vinaigrette as a dipping sauce for fresh vegetables. ≈

Day 13

The Real You

You made all the delicate, inner parts of my body and knit me together in my mother's womb. Thank you for making me so wonderfully complex! Your workmanship is marvelous—how well I know it.

Psalm 139:13–14 (NLT)

You were made by God. You were knit together by the hands of God. Have you ever knitted or watched someone else knit? I have an aunt who loves to knit. She always has her knitting needles and yarn in her hands. She is always creating an item with her own special touch that makes each piece beautifully unique. That is how God made each of us, with His special touch that created each of us beautifully unique.

When my aunt knits, a single strand of yarn is continuously pulled into, around, and through, creating complex patterns and resulting in an amazing creation. And what is our response to her creations? "That's gorgeous!" is our reply as we stand in awe of her talented workmanship. Our Heavenly Father has done the same with us. He has knitted together delicate parts to create an astonishing, complex creation—YOU!

God's most marvelous workmanship is not the Grand Canyon or Mount Everest—it's YOU. Yet we find it so difficult to think of ourselves as marvelous. We live in a world where we are constantly told we are not good enough, thin enough, or talented enough, and we start to believe that this is who we really are. But God's Word tells us that we are wonderfully complex and a marvelous work of God's hands. So how do we choose to believe God's Truth about who we really are instead of what the world is throwing at us? We begin by thanking God for making us wonderfully complex and unique. We praise Him for His marvelous workmanship in creating us. When we do this continually, thanking and praising God for the Truth about ourselves that we find in His Word, we nurture a heart full of gratitude that believes and knows, "I am wonderful and marvelous because God has made me that way."

Taking It to Heart

1. How does it feel to know that God's hand made every part of your body and mind?

2. How would you live differently if you fully believed that you are wonderful and marvelous?

Day 13 ~ The Real You

3. What is stopping you from living that way?

4. What can you do to remove that roadblock?

Heavenly Father and Daughter Time

Spend time thanking God for making you wonderful, marvelous, and beautiful. Praise Him for His marvelous workmanship in creating you.

Temple Tip for the Day

Replace your scale with a tape measure! ≈

Day 14

Am I Beautiful?

Do you believe you are beautiful? Can you look at yourself in the mirror and think, "I am beautiful"? For some women, answering yes to that question might be easy, but for me it was almost impossible to say, "Yes, I am beautiful."

For most of my life I defined beauty by looking to the beauty icons and fashion gurus of the world. And when I compared myself to those standards I came up short every time, which just made me feel ugly and undesirable. Then I became a Christian and I learned that God defines beauty very differently than the world.

> *Don't be concerned about the outward beauty of fancy hairstyles, expensive jewelry, or beautiful clothes. You should clothe yourselves instead with the beauty that comes from within, the unfading beauty of a gentle and quiet spirit, which is so precious to God. This is how the holy women of old made themselves beautiful. They put their trust in God.*
>
> 1 Peter 3:3–5 (NLT)

When I first read this scripture I was drawn to the idea that God finds a gentle and quiet spirit precious and beautiful. In fact, that is His definition of beauty. But this idea did not bring me comfort or make me feel beautiful. I struggled with the words *gentle* and *quiet* because I am a high-energy person with a not-so-quiet voice. In fact, early in my marriage my husband would often say to me, "Why are you yelling?" To me I wasn't yelling, I was just talking, but to him the volume of my voice was the equivalent of yelling. This is just proof that I am not a quiet person.

Day 14 ~ Am I Beautiful?

OK, so now not only did I not measure up to the world's standard of beauty, but I also did not measure up to God's standard of beauty. Ugh!!! My frustration came from defining God's standard of beauty with the world's interpretation and not with the understanding of the Holy Spirit. So I read that scripture again.

First I saw that 1 Peter says, "a gentle and quiet *spirit,* not voice or personality. Then I took a closer look at the words *gentle* and *quiet.* To be gentle means not to be insistent or demand your own way, not to be pushy and selfishly assertive. In the book *Girls Gone Wise in a World Gone Wild,* author Mary Kassian says, "Calmness is the second characteristic. Most translations use the word quiet to describe this attitude of serenity and tranquility. Being calm means being settled, firm, immovable, steadfast and peaceful in spirit. A calm disposition is like a still, peaceful pool of water, as opposed to a churning whirlpool that's agitated and stirred up." Later she says that "quietness has more to do with the state of our hearts than the quantity and volume of our words."

So the volume of our voice, the number of words we speak, and our personalities are not the dictating factors in whether or not we have a gentle and calm spirit. A gentle and calm spirit is the heart motive that drives the voice, the words, and the personality. Our heart is the guiding compass behind our voice and personality. For me this was good news: I could be outgoing and strong and passionate while also possessing a quiet and gentle spirit underneath. That said, it's also important to note that a woman can be shy and quiet while possessing a rebellious and bitter spirit. Wow, we really can't judge a book by its cover.

So how do we nurture this kind of heart motive? As verse 5 says, we learn from examples who came before us, from those who put their trust in the Lord. Look at the women of the Bible, our mothers, our grandmothers, women in our church, and others who have placed their trust in God and live with a heart of gentleness and quietness. These examples teach us that the best way to develop a gentle and quiet spirit is to develop our relationship with God. The more we get to know Him, the more we see His unfailing love for us, His promises for our future, and His faithfulness through out history. When we grow in our knowledge of God, we learn we can trust Him, which allows the fruit of gentleness to grow in us. We can't do it without God. This doesn't mean we are not also to take care of the outside. We are to care for His temple. But make sure your priority is your relationship with the Lord. As this relationship strengthens and deepens with time, it will nurture a beauty that never fades.

Now, if you are anything like me, at this point you might be saying, "Sure, having a gentle and quiet spirit will make me beautiful, but I still think my butt's too big or my nose is a funny shape or I need to lose 10 pounds." I know, I get it: our bodies are not perfect—but according to whom? When we put ourselves down and point out what we think is wrong with us, we are telling God that His creation is ugly and not good enough.

So God created human beings in his own image. In the image of God he created them; male and female he created them.

Genesis 1:27 (NLT)

We are made in the image of God. Do you believe that God is ugly? If not, then you can only conclude that because you believe that God is beautiful and you are made like Him, then you also are beautiful. And those who speak against that Truth, including us, are speaking lies.

Taking It to Heart

1. To you, what does a woman look like who possesses a gentle and quiet spirit?

Day 14 ~ Am I Beautiful?

2. On a scale of 1 to 7 (with 1 being the worst and 7 being the best), how do you rate the development of your own "gentle spirit"?

3. On a scale of 1 to 7, how do you rate the development of your "quiet spirit"?

4. If your answers are not 7, what would it take to get them to 7?

5. What next step could you take to move toward a 7 for a gentle and quiet spirit?

6. When will you take that next step?

Heavenly Father and Daughter Time

Confess any lies that you have been speaking against God's Truth that you are beautiful, and ask that He renew a gentle and quiet spirit within you.

Temple Tip for the Day

Create make-and-go snack packs filled with healthy foods such as nuts, seeds, fruits, and sliced veggies. Take them with you on busy days so that you avoid unhealthy temptations. ≈

Day 15

Addicted

It's confession time! Hello, my name is Lisa and I am addicted to sugar. Anyone else want to stand up and take a turn at confessing a food you can't live without? Let's be honest: sometimes it's hard to tell if we are addicted or just enjoy food a lot. But here's one example of how I knew I had an addiction. When my husband would leave for work in the morning, I would get in my car and drive to the local grocery store and purchase donuts—two, three, or sometimes four. I would do this several times a week. I would come home, eat breakfast, maybe some eggs or cereal, and then I would dive into those donuts, eating 2 or 3 right after breakfast. I wasn't hungry, I just wanted to eat those donuts. It gave me great pleasure at the time, but later I would feel terrible about what I had done. If I didn't eat all the donuts I purchased that day, I would hide them in the pantry where my husband would not see them so I could have them later in the day or the next morning after he was gone. And that is how I discovered my addiction: I hid food from my husband so that he wouldn't know I was eating it. I didn't want to give in to my craving for those donuts, but I just couldn't stop. I knew there was something wrong in the fact that I was hiding food from my husband, but I still couldn't stop. I became a slave to my craving.

Food addiction, or in my case sugar addiction, is not a myth, nor should it be taken lightly. In our brain is a "reward system" designed to "reward" our body when we do things that encourage our survival, such as eating. Our brain then releases feel-good chemicals, including a neurotransmitter called dopamine, which our brains interpret as pleasure. We are hardwired to seek out behaviors that release dopamine. The problem is we get a more powerful release of dopamine when we eat "junk food" than when we eat a steak or a carrot. When we eat foods that repeatedly release these massive amounts of dopamine, our brain recognizes that the levels are too high and it lowers the output to keep us balanced. When you have fewer receptors you start to feel unhappy if you don't get your "fix," and you need more dopamine to feel the same effect as before, which means you will eat even more junk food. We become addicted to the junk food because we want to feel that same pleasurable high. (From www.authoritynutrition.com.)

I don't share this information in order to create an excuse for us, but rather to help us become more aware of how our bodies work, and about the role that God plays in breaking our addictions. God is the One who designed our brain to enjoy the food He has prepared for us to eat in order to survive. But it is we who have chosen to use food to seek pleasure and we are entertained and satisfied by that pleasure. And this is how we become a slave to food: we believe we "need" a certain food and deserve a certain food, and we crave that certain food to make us feel satisfied and happy, and if we don't get it we feel sad and deprived. We thus fall into a trap of believing that food is for pleasure, and we keep seeking that pleasure until it controls our behavior—like me hiding food in my own house in my determination to satisfy my craving.

But here is the good news!

Don't you realize that you become the slave of whatever you choose to obey? You can be a slave to sin, which leads to death, or you can choose to obey God, which leads to righteous living.

Romans 6:16 (NLT)

You can choose! You can choose to follow your own cravings, which leads to feelings of disappointment in yourself for giving in to the craving, and then to unhappiness and addiction. And sometimes our food addictions lead to eating disorders such as binge eating, bulimia, or anorexia. Or you can choose to follow God and His design for good health. There are some who have a serious food addiction and need to seek professional help through a counselor or a local food-addiction group such as Overeaters Anonymous. But for most of us it comes down to a choice: follow our own sinful desires and be a slave, or follow God and be free!

> *Thank God! Once you were slaves of sin, but now you wholeheartedly obey this teaching we have given you. Now you are free from your slavery to sin, and you have become slaves to righteous living.*
>
> *Romans 6:17–18 (NLT)*

Thank God, because without Jesus we would not have a choice, but because of Him we can choose God as our master. We can't break our addiction without Jesus. We must wholeheartedly give ourselves fully to God, and that includes what we eat. If we love God with all our heart, mind, and soul, He becomes our master and shapes our thoughts and attitudes about food. In our times of cravings and overwhelming desires we must turn to Him, because He is the only one who can break our addiction to food. He is the only one who can give us freedom from the food that has enslaved us and is controlling our choices.

Taking It to Heart

1. What "junk food" do you feel you are addicted to?

2. How do you feel when you give in to a craving for that food?

3. Do you like feeling that way?

4. How can you allow God to help you when you are faced with the tempting craving for that food?

5. How will you remember to take that step?

Heavenly Father and Daughter Time

Confess to your Heavenly Father your food addiction, its control over you, and how it has made you a slave to sinful ways. Accept His forgiveness and rejoice that you are breaking free from food controlling you ever again.

Temple Tip for the Day

Remember that food is meant to nourish our bodies, not entertain our minds! ≈

Day 16

The Feeding Trough

Where I live we have a restaurant that we affectionately call "the feeding trough." It is an all-you-can-eat smorgasbord restaurant with enough food options and quantities to feed a small country. We would go there on my birthday because the birthday person always eats for free. What could be more glorious than eating all you want for free! They place your party at a table, then you head to the buffet and fill your plate with as many savory samples as it will hold, only to return later and fill another plate, and then another plate. Of course let's not forget about the dessert buffet. But by then you are so full that one plate full of sweets will suffice.

Upon leaving "the feeding trough" I would be stuffed to the max and feeling like my pants had somehow shrunk a size during my visit. But everything tasted so good, so I would endure how physically uncomfortable I was and tolerate how sluggish I felt as I digested all that food. I would justify my trip to "the feeding trough" by using the excuse that I didn't do this all the time, so it's OK to do it every once in a while. Oh how I wish that were true. Upon further examination of my eating habits, I discovered that this was NOT the only time I overate.

Have you ever eaten a meal that was so good you just wanted to have a little bit more,but you weren't really hungry, you just wanted to savor that yummy food one more time? Or after finishing a satisfying dinner have you reached for dessert not because you needed it but because of course you *must* have that sweet after your meal? Or did you decide to eat just one meal a day—a meal that began in the morning and ended at bedtime? You are constantly putting food in your mouth whether you are hungry or not because you like the taste and you want it. When taste overrules hunger and our want outweighs our need, we have moved into the territory of eating in excess. Excessive eating is called gluttony. I'm sure most of us have heard of gluttony before, but have we ever recognized that gluttony is a sin?

Make no mistake, the Bible is clear that gluttony is a sin. But we Christians do a great job of ignoring this fact. We don't talk about it, we don't usually hear a sermon on the subject, and most of us don't want to admit that our eating habits are an offense to God. But *all* sin is an offense to God. So why is this sin of gluttony so easily ignored, dismissed, and excused? Here is what the Bible has to say about the sin of gluttony:

> *O my son, be wise and stay in God's paths; don't carouse with drunkards and gluttons, for they are on their way to poverty. And remember that too much sleep clothes a man with rags.*
>
> *Proverbs 23:19–21 (TLB)*

> *A discerning son heeds instruction, but a companion of gluttons disgraces his father.*
>
> *Proverbs 28:7 (NIV)*

> *"The Son of Man, on the other hand, feasts and drinks, and you say, 'He's a glutton and a drunkard, and a friend of tax collectors and other sinners!'"*
>
> *Matthew 11:19 (NLT)*

> *Even one of their own men, a prophet from Crete, has said about them, "The people of Crete are all liars, cruel animals, and lazy gluttons."*
>
> *Titus 1:12 (NLT)*

In these examples from scripture we can see that we are advised not to hang out with or be a companion of gluttons because being a glutton leads to poverty, meaning that others' gluttony is an undesirable quality that could influence us to be the same and bring disgrace. Being a glutton is associated with laziness and that is not pleasing to God. In Matthew 11, *glutton* was one accusation thrown at Jesus to discredit Him, showing us that gluttony was considered a sin by the Jews.

With such a clear understanding that gluttony is a sin, I again wonder, why do we Christians so easily dismiss the Truth and make excuses about our sin of gluttony? I believe the answer is that we have chosen to ignore it and have grown accustomed to living in a world of excess. Because we need food to survive, eating becomes a balancing act between moderation and excess. In the scriptures quoted above, gluttony is mentioned alongside drunkenness to show us that just like drinking alcohol is not in itself a sin and must be done in moderation in order to avoid the sin of drunkenness, food also must be consumed in moderation to avoid the sin of gluttony. We live in a world of excess, never satisfied with the portions we are given. We want more! We want what we want when we want it, and then we want more of it. But we are not called to live like the world; we are called to be an example of balance and moderation.

> *But the fruit of the Spirit is love, joy, peace, patience, kindness, goodness, faithfulness, gentleness, self-control; against such things there is no law.*
> *Galatians 5:22–23 (NIV)*

Moderation is achieved through self-control, a product of God working in us. It's interesting that the term *self-control* is not about our "self" having control and cannot be produced by the self. Rather, it is produced when we give up our control, allow God to renew our mind and heart with His Truth, and choose to follow His teachings. When we can't control our appetite, it is an indication that a spiritual problem is taking place, and that problem is lack of self-control. We can live a balanced life of moderation if we choose to rely solely on His strength to help us control our appetite. We can't do it on our own!

Taking It to Heart

1. Examine your eating habits. Are you choosing to overeat?

2. Why are you choosing to eat more even when you are not hungry?

3. What step could you take not to overeat?

Day 16 ~ The Feeding Trough

4. What might hinder you from taking that step?

5. How can you minimize that hindrance?

Heavenly Father and Daughter Time

Seek forgiveness from your Heavenly Father for your sin of gluttony. Ask Him to help you control your appetite.

Temple Tip for the Day

When you pray before each meal, include asking God to help you control your portion size and to give you discernment between hunger and want. ≈

Day 17

Habit vs. Hunger

When we watch movies we eat popcorn. When we have a campfire we make and eat s'mores. When we have dinner we have dessert. Before bedtime we have a snack. Do any of these scenarios sound familiar to you? They are all familiar to me, because they are some of my favorite eating habits. But that's all they are:habits. They are eating choices that have turned into patterns that have become almost involuntary. They are not eating choices made because I was hungry, but eating choices made without even thinking about it and doing it because that is what I have always done. Now, I am not saying that any of these eating choices are bad (when you are *not* on the fast). However, I am challenged by the question, are we honoring God's temple when we make eating choices on the basis of involuntary responses to certain cues in our lives? For example, the cue is watching a movie, the involuntary response is eating popcorn, and the result is a habit.

The question then is, are these habits nourishing the body or trashing the temple? To answer that question, let's consider our heart motives for making these eating choices. For what is in a woman's heart influences what she thinks and how she acts.

> *Therefore, I urge you, brothers, in view of God's mercy, to offer your bodies as living sacrifices, holy and pleasing to God—this is your spiritual act of worship. Do not conform to the pattern of this world, but be transformed by the renewing of your mind. Then you will be able to test and approve what God's will is—his good, pleasing and perfect will.*
>
> *Romans 12:1–2 (NIV)*

Day 17 ~ Habit vs. Hunger

In this scripture, Paul is asking us to offer ourselves as a living sacrifice, meaning that each day we surrender our desires and wants and live a life devoted to serving and pleasing God as an act of worshipping the One who sacrificed His only Son so that we can be forgiven for our sins. Through Christ we have been set free of the punishment we deserve—that is God's mercy. Our response to such a great gift should be gratitude. And when our heart motive is one of gratitude, we will be compelled to do those things that are pleasing to God and bring Him honor and glory.

How does a heart motive of gratitude help us to recognize and change a poor eating habit? We need to allow God to change our thinking so we can recognize the difference between the behaviors and customs of this world—that is, our poor eating habits—and His good, pleasing, and perfect will for us. When our thinking is changed, our habits can be transformed.

How do we change our thinking?

Set your minds on things above, not on earthly things.

Colossians 3:2 (NIV)

To "set your mind on things above" is to intentionally seek God in order to learn His ways. We renew our minds daily by being in His Word and communicating with our Heavenly Father. When we learn His ways and His desires, we equip our hearts and minds with His Truth, and then we can compare our habits to His Truth to see if what we are doing is pleasing to God and will bring us good health and a prosperous soul.

Taking It to Heart

Steps to recognizing if we are nourishing the body or trashing the temple:

1. *Heart motive:* remember all that God has done for you and allow that Truth to compel you to choose eating habits that bring Him honor and glory.

2. *Question:* Bring each habit before God and His Truth. Thoughtfully and prayerfully consider if you are choosing this food because you are hungry or because it is a habit, then wait for the answer. Compare your choice to God's desire that you have good health and a prosperous soul.

3. *Do not conform:* If your habit is trashing the temple, choose to stop doing it.

4. *Renew your mind:* Continue in His Word and allow Him to align your thinking with His Truth.

5. *Transformed:* Continue in the previous steps until you are no longer mindless in your food choices and your actions in choosing food demonstrate your grateful heart and bring God honor and glory.

Heavenly Father and Daughter Time

Ask your Heavenly Father to help you recognize those eating habits that are trashing your body, His temple.

Temple Tip for the Day

Keep a food journal. Write down what and when you eat. This will help you to recognize the eating habits that are not bringing you good health and a prosperous soul. ≈

Day 18

Running For Comfort

Why am I eating this? That's the question I asked myself as I grabbed another candy bar that day. I had found myself stuck in a pattern in which I felt helpless. I was feeling stressed out about getting the house cleaned, working, and preparing food for a dinner party we were having the next day. And in my moment of feeling overwhelmed, what did I do to find relief? I ate another candy bar. As soon as I ate it I felt relieved of the stress, but that relief was shortly followed by guilt because it was my third candy bar of the day.

I guess that wouldn't be so bad if it was just that one day. But the more I looked at why and when and what I was eating, the more God revealed a deeper issue in my heart. I began to notice that when I was feeling stressed, depressed, overwhelmed, sad, lonely, bored, hurt, or irritated, I would run to the pantry to find relief from those emotions. I don't like feeling those emotions, and I craved comfort for those negative feelings. So I ran to food to comfort my soul. I did that so often that eventually I believed I needed food to comfort me.

But the comfort I received from food was not comfort at all but merely a means to ignore what my emotions where trying to tell me. God designed us to be emotional creatures—to feel all emotions: love, joy, sadness, loneliness, hurt, and so on. He gave us emotions as indicators, to let us know when something is good or when something is wrong. So by eating to subdue my negative emotions, I inevitably stuffed my problems with food and numbed my heart to the solution, and that is not comfort at all.

> *Praise be to the God and Father of our Lord Jesus Christ, the Father of compassion and the God of all comfort, who comforts us in all our troubles.*
> *2 Corinthians 1:3–4 (NIV)*

Our emotions tell us when we are having trouble, and in that trouble we run for comfort. We run for a sense of relief, to be encouraged, find help, and be strengthened. That's what true comfort is. God gave us our emotional indicators of trouble so that in our effort to find comfort we would run to Him, the God of all comfort and the One who promises to give us comfort in all trouble. God promises to be our strength, we find encouragement and help in His Word, and through prayer we gain a sense of relief. Food cannot make those promises. But not using food to stuff down my negative emotions means I have to feel them and deal with the root cause, and that scared me.

> *For God did not give us a spirit of timidity, but a spirit of power, of love and of self-discipline.*
> *2 Timothy 1:7 (NIV)*

Not only did God design us to be emotional, but He also gave us a spirit of power, love, and self-discipline, not a spirit of fear. We don't have to be afraid to feel the negative emotions or face the root cause of them. The Truth is that the Holy Spirit living within us gives us the power to break the bondage of emotional eating by giving us courage and self-desciplne to face the root of our negative emotions and choose to find comfort in our Heavenly Father's arms.

Taking It to Heart

1. What emotion are you experiencing that makes you want to eat?

2. What is the root or cause of that emotion?

3. Will eating solve your problem?

4. Will eating create a new problem or emotion? Explain.

5. What do you think God wants to teach you through this trouble?

6. How can running to God give you comfort in this time of trouble?

Heavenly Father and Daughter Time

Spend time telling your Heavenly Father about your current troubles, ask for His help and strength to face the cause of the trouble, and be still and receive His comfort.

Temple Tip for the Day

Before eating, stop and ask yourself, "Why am I eating this?" We should be eating to nourish our bodies, not to hide our troubles. ≈

Day 19

My Two Best Friends: Guilt and Shame

In the summer of 1999 I found myself standing alone in my bathroom holding onto a white plastic stick that read *pregnant!* I was single and had been dating this guy only a couple of months. My mind raced with thoughts like, What will my Christian parents think? What will my friends say? How am I going to tell my boyfriend and what will his reaction be? I felt so scared and alone. When I told my boyfriend, his reaction to the news was first anger, then telling me all the reasons I shouldn't have the baby—reasons like "We can't afford to have this child," "I can't afford the 3 children I already have," and "You wouldn't be a good mother to bring a child into this situation." And he made it clear that if I were to have this child, I couldn't depend on him for anything. My mind was already overwhelmed with thoughts of how disappointed my parents and friends would be in me, and now my heart was breaking with the feeling of possibly losing a love I had just found. So I decided to have an abortion. What I thought was an easy solution to my problem of being pregnant became the invitation for guilt and shame to become my best friends.

Even though I believed what the world taught—that abortion was not wrong and was merely a woman's choice—I woke up from the procedure with a sense of devastating regret and a heart wound oozing with guilt and shame. The pain of that guilt and shame over what I had done was too great to bear, so I hid it deep within my heart. The problem with hiding our guilt and shame is that they don't disappear but instead manifest themselves in different forms. My unresolved guilt and shame over what I had done resurfaced as depression. Then later, when I became a Christian, they appeared as fear that someone would find out what I had done and reject me.

Since the beginning of time, mankind has been trying to hide our sinful acts from God. As soon as Adam and Eve ate from the tree from which God had commanded them not to eat, they felt guilt and shame, covered themselves with fig leaves, and "hid themselves from the Lord God among the trees of the garden" (Genesis 3:8 NIV). But God saw and knew exactly what they had done. How silly they were to think that they could hide from an all-knowing, all-seeing God behind a few fig leaves and a couple of trees. Yet that is exactly what we do. We act like we can cover up what we are doing and thus hide from God our guilt and shame over what we have done. But God has given us the feelings of guilt and shame not to condemn us but to make us aware of our sin so that we can confess it and receive forgiveness.

> *If we confess our sins, God is faithful and righteous to forgive us our sins and to cleanse us from all unrighteousness.*
>
> 1 John 1:9 (HCSB)

> *Therefore, there is now no condemnation for those who are in Christ Jesus.*
>
> Romans 8:1 (NIV)

When I chose to stop hiding my guilt and shame over having an abortion and allowed those emotions to bring me to Jesus, I confessed before Him what I had done and received His forgiveness, and now I live a life free from condemnation—a life free from guilt, shame, and my sin of abortion! There is no sin that is so great that God cannot forgive it, but all sin produces feelings of guilt and shame, and God wants to resolve those feelings. Let them drive you toward the cross, where you can find forgiveness and freedom.[1]

---

[1] If you are a post-abortive woman who has not yet gone through a healing journey for your abortion and you desire to know more about that, please contact us at www.revealredeemrestore.com.

Day 19 ~ My Two Best Friends

Taking It to Heart

1. What sin are you hiding that is producing guilt and shame in your life?

2. Why are you hiding it?

3. Read 1 John 1:9 again. Do you believe that God is faithful and will forgive that sin when you confess it to Him?

4. Do you desire freedom from your feelings of guilt and shame?

Heavenly Father and Daughter Time

Confess any unresolved sin in your life. Then ask for and receive God's forgiveness for that sin. Thank God for His faithfulness in cleansing you of your guilt and shame.

Temple Tip of the Day

Enjoy your newfound freedom of guilt and shame in a special way! For example, take a Praise-Filled Power Walk around your neighborhood, or get creative; just don't use food as your reward. ≈

Day 20

Unraveling Anger

Have you ever noticed that when you show anger, people seem to think you are being ungodly? Or you are told you shouldn't be angry because that doesn't solve anything. Or people believe that if you are angry you are a bad person. But did you know that God tells us to be angry?!

> *Be angry, and yet do not sin; do not let the sun go down on your anger.*
>
> *Ephesians 4:26 (NASB)*

As believers, we must be careful not to confuse anger the emotion with anger set in motion as sin. Anger is a God-given response to when we are betrayed or hurt, feel fear or are attacked, experience injustice or selfish ambition. But feeling angry is not a sin; it is what we do with it that is either a sinful response or a God-honoring response.

I have a good friend who always says that our choices can either bring us life (spiritual freedom) or bring us death (spiritual consequences of sin). There are two stories from the Bible that show us anger bringing life and anger bringing death.

One day after Moses had risen to a position of great influence in Pharaoh's house, he witnessed an Egyptian beating a Hebrew slave, one of his own people. Moses grew angry, looked around to make sure no one saw him, and killed the Egyptian and buried him in the sand. The next day he saw two Hebrews fighting and questioned why they were attacking each other. One of the men replied to Moses, "Who made you ruler and judge over us? Are you thinking of killing me as you did the Egyptian?" Moses became afraid because what he had done was not a secret, and he had to flee because Pharaoh found out what he had done and tried to kill him (Exodus 2:11–15 NIV). Moses had every right to be angry about the injustice he had witnessed against his people. But his response to his anger was to secretly take matters into his own hands and cast judgment, enact punishment, and seek revenge for himself. His anger response was motivated by selfish desires and resulted in sin.

The other story is of Jesus entering the temple and seeing the businessmen cheating and exploiting those who had come to worship, and he grew angry. He overturned tables, drove out those who were buying and selling animals for sacrifice, and said to them, "The scriptures declare, 'My temple will be called a house of prayer, but you have turned it into a den of thieves' " (Matthew 21:12–16 NLT). Jesus too demonstrated anger, but His anger response was not sin, first because there is no sin in Him, and second because His motive was not selfish like Moses's was; instead his response was out of love for those who came to worship God and find healing.

Now, I know these are two extreme examples of responses to anger, but they demonstrate clearly that we need to check our motives when we act out our anger. God did not give us anger so that we can damage relationships; he gave us anger to reveal the root emotion so that we can deal with it in an appropriate way. Our goal in dealing with anger should always be healing for ourselves and helping others and our relationships. We do this by not letting anger control our actions.

> *Don't sin by letting anger control you. Think about it overnight and remain silent.*
> *Psalm 4:4 (NLT)*

When anger controls us, we respond with a sinful attitude or action that might cause damage to ourselves or others emotionally, physically, and spiritually. So God challenges us to pause in our anger, to think about it and be silent overnight so that we don't react irrationally but rather allow ourselves time to process the root emotion of our anger and respond in a way that is God-honoring.

Day 20 ~ Unraveling Anger

I don't know about you but sometimes I just feel like if I don't release my anger I will explode, and not in a good way. This is why God tells us, "do not let the sun go down on your anger." He tells us this because He understands that we must do something with our anger. There are healthy ways to deal with anger. During the healing journey for the post-abortive women I work with we address healthy ways to release anger. One activity we have them do is write an "angry letter" to the person or circumstance with which they are angry. They do not send or give these letters to anyone; rather, they write the letters to release the anger, then we tear them up and burn them in the fire pit in my back yard.

Be angry, discover the root of your anger, and release your anger in a healthy way so that your response will bring God honor, which brings healing and forgiveness to you and your relationships.

Taking It to Heart

1. Who or what are you angry with?

2. What emotion is the root of your anger?

3. How have you responded to your anger? Has it been God honoring or sinful?

Heavenly Father and Daughter Time

If you have allowed anger to control you and enacted a sinful response, ask God to forgive your response. Ask your Heavenly Father to heal the emotion at the root of your anger and show you how to respond in a God-honoring way.

Temple Tip for the Day

Write an "angry letter" to the person or circumstance with which you are angry. Don't hold back! Write down everything you want to release. Do not send it or read it to another person. Now tear it up and throw it away or burn it to release your anger, and as you do this say, "I'm letting go of my anger toward you. I choose to forgive you so that I may be healed from this burden of anger." ≈

Day 21

Forgiveness Is NOT a Feeling

The man I was dating when I had an abortion was, I believed, the "man of my dreams," but he turned out to be a nightmare. He became abusive, first emotionally, then financially, and finally physically. He moved us far away from my family and friends, and there the abuse got worse. With the help of family I got out of that situation, and shortly thereafter I gave my life to Christ.

When I gave my life to Christ I knew He forgave me for my sins, but there was no way I could forgive myself for having an abortion, and I definitely didn't feel like I needed to forgive that man for all the horrible things he did to me. But because I felt like I couldn't forgive myself, and because I didn't feel like my abuser deserved forgiveness, I created a foothold for Satan, a place where the enemy securely planted his feet and began to poison my mind with his lies and enslave my heart with anger and bitterness.

In 2006 I went on a healing journey for my wound of abortion and there is where I finally surrendered to God my sin of abortion and the condemning lies I believed. And when I fully accepted *His* truth that "He forgives all your sins and does not treat you as your sins deserve" (Psalm 103:3, 10, NIV), *my* life was set free. It was like being set free from a prison cell and leaving behind the guilt, shame, and condemnation, never to be imprisoned again for my offenses.

So to me forgiveness is about freedom—*my* freedom. Through my experience in forgiving myself I learned about the benefits of forgiving others. When I choose to forgive it does not mean I forget; it means I don't hold on to the offense and then use it later against the offender. It does not minimize the offense either. Choosing to forgive my abuser doesn't mean that what he did was excusable; it means that I am not holding on to the possibility of revenge. Ultimately, forgiveness sets me and you free from the bondage of anger and bitterness.

I once heard someone use this quote: "Holding on to unforgiveness is like me drinking poison and waiting for the other person to die." I don't know who said it originally but I laugh every time I hear it, then realize the truth in it. We believe the lie that if we stay angry and refuse to forgive our offender, somehow we are punishing that person. But if we as Christ followers say, "I know God forgives me but I can't forgive myself or I can't forgive that person," we elevate our ability to forgive over God's. So the truth is that our unforgiveness becomes our offense against God.

Make allowances for each other's faults, and forgive anyone who offends you. Remember, the Lord forgave you, so you must forgive others.

Colossians 3:13 (NLT)

So forgiveness is not about us waiting to feel like we are ready to forgive the offender; it is about choosing to act in obedience to God's command to forgive others. It was a difficult choice to forgive someone who had abused me. I had to surrender my anger toward him and my desire for revenge. But when we surrender those things and choose to forgive, we set our hearts free and demonstrate to others the joy and peace of knowing God's forgiveness.

Taking It to Heart

1. Are you holding on to unforgiveness toward someone or yourself?

2. How is holding onto unforgiveness affecting your joy and peace?

3. Do you believe that we are to forgive others just as the Lord has forgiven us?

4. Are you ready to choose to forgive that person or those persons, yourself, or both so that your heart may be free of anger and bitterness?

Heavenly Father and Daughter Time

Write the name(s) of the person(s) you are choosing to forgive on a piece of paper. Pray to release all anger, bitterness, vengefulness, and unforgiveness. Allow the peace of Christ to fill your heart. Tear up the paper with the name(s) on it and throw it away as you pray these words: "I am tossing my unforgiveness away so that I may be free."

Temple Tip of the Day

Try to make 60 percent or more of your intake raw foods. Eat live, raw food with every meal. ≈

Day 22

Portion Distortion

I have heard the phrase *portion control* used as a reminder to be attentive to the serving size of the food we eat at meals and in snacks. I know the intention is to make us aware that we are in control of the size and frequency of the portions we choose to eat. What I found is that I had *complete* control over the portion size of the foods I ate. I had control over the large amount of food I would plop onto my plate, including the size of the second helping I would take if it was really yummy. I was the one in control of choosing to snack on a few handfuls of chips or to follow a meal with a few scoops of ice cream. It was always my choice how much I ate. You see, my problem wasn't portion control at all but rather my assumption that the amount I was eating was OK and the correct serving size for a meal or snack. Thus I was operating under "portion distortion"!

Portion distortion is when we assume that the amount of food we serve ourselves and are served in restaurants as a portion for one person is correct. Seventy percent of Americans who responded to a recent poll by the Mollen Foundation felt that the amount of food we eat at home and the amount we are served at restaurants are "normal" serving sizes. What we have failed to realize is that portion sizes have increased over the years. For example, 20 years ago a bagel was 3 inches in diameter and 140 calories, but today bagels are an average of 6 inches in diameter and 350 calories. And there is a difference between "portion size" and "serving size." A portion is a person's own choice of how much to put on her plate and in her mouth, and because it is a choice it will vary from person to person, so we need a standard to guide us, and that standard is called the serving size. A serving size is an estab-

Day 22 ~ Portion Distortion

lished measurement of food, such as a cup or an ounce. Why, then, do we have portion distortion?

All a man's ways seem right to him, but the Lord weighs the heart.

Proverbs 21:2 (NIV)

We have portion distortion because we believe the size and frequency of the portions we choose are correct when in fact they are not. Whether we choose an oversized portion or a second helping or decide to eat a little less, we have a false sense of portion control because we are relying on what we think is right. Because the choice of our portion size will always be in our control, and because our choices come from our motives, our motives should be about bringing God glory and not about pleasing ourselves.

So whether you eat or drink, or whatever you do, do it all for the glory of God.

1 Corinthians 10:31 (NLT)

I can honestly say that in the past when I was deciding how much to eat or drink, my motive was not to bring glory to God. But if I love God, then all I do, including what and how much I eat, is motivated by that love. My love for God is my portion control.

You, Lord, are my choice and I will obey you.

Psalm 119:57 (CEV)

I say: The Lord is my portion, therefore I will put my hope in Him.

Lamentations 3:24 (HCSB)

When we choose God, we do so because of His great love for us and out of our love for Him, and that love compels us to want to obey Him. But overeating, being addicted to food, and eating to stuff my emotions are not choices that bring God glory. My heart was also operating under portion distortion, meaning I was choosing to seek satisfaction, comfort, and peace in food instead of seeking the Lord and being obedient in caring for His Temple.

Obeying God is not about denying ourselves the portion; it's about the portion itself. *Portion* means enough and *having enough* means we are satisfied. So, when we say that the Lord is our portion we are saying that the Lord is enough and we are satisfied in Him. I don't need to look to a heaping portion of food to sooth my soul or comfort my emotions, because the Lord is the portion that brings me comfort, peace, and hope.

Portion control is our choice. A serving size of God is the portion that will fill us, satisfy us, comfort us, and free us from our addiction to food and our desire to overeat, if we choose it.

Taking It to Heart

1. How have your eating habits and heart motives been under a portion distortion?

2. How would being satisfied and full of God change your choices of what and how much you eat and drink?

Day 22 ~ Portion Distortion

3. Describe how your choices of what you eat and drink can bring God glory.

4. What changes do you need to make to your eating and drinking habits in order to bring God glory?

Heavenly Father and Daughter Time

Seek the fullness of God by choosing Him as your portion. Allow your time with Him to be the serving size you need in order not to run to food for comfort, peace, and hope.

Temple Tip for the Day

The best way to determine the amount of food in a serving is to measure it out. Read the label or a reliable source for recommended serving sizes and measure out that amount to see the correct portion size. ≈

Day 23

The Scale of Bondage

In the past when I set out on a weight-loss journey I would measure my success by how many pounds I lost. Each week I would slowly move toward the scale and with an anxious heart I would step on it and watch the numbers rise. I could feel my emotions shift from excitement to disappointment as I watched the numbers bounce around that little red line that was about to land on the number that decided my fate. If I had lost pounds, I felt pleased with myself and was encouraged to keep moving forward and I might celebrate with a "little" treat. If I had gained any amount of weight, I felt completely discouraged and would give up, thinking why bother, I'm never going to lose weight. I measured my success by the outcome on that scale and allowed those numbers to determine how I felt about myself and my body. I allowed the scale to control my emotions and actions. I was in bondage to the scale.

For you are a slave to whatever controls you.

2 Peter 2:19 (NLT)

A slave is bound to a master. That master dictates our actions and dominates our life. I had placed the scale in a position of great authority; it was my master when it came to how I felt about my body and weight-loss success or failure. But when I became a Christian I chose to allow God to be my master, and scripture teaches that "no one can serve two masters" (Matthew 6:24, NIV). I needed to decide what was going to dominate my life—a scale or God and His Truth.

Before I made that decision I wanted to know why I had made the scale my master to begin with. What the Holy Spirit revealed to me at that time was that I had manufactured in my mind an ideal of what my weight should be and I had accepted an untrue image of beauty. I had made an idol.

> *How foolish are those who manufacture idols. These prized objects are really worthless. The people who worship idols don't know this, so they are all put to shame.*
> *Isaiah 44:9 (NLT)*

Whatever we allow to go into our minds, through our eyes and ears, will determine our thoughts and actions. My source of beauty and acceptable weight was images of movie stars, celebrities, advertisements, and the fashion industry. I allowed the standards of this world to become my idol, and that idol transferred onto my scale, which became my master in deciding how I felt about myself and my body, which I thought was ugly and worthless.

But then I decided to allow God's Truth to break my scale bondage and to allow God to be the master of my life. So the first thing I did was to "flee from idolatry" (1 Corinthians 10:14, NIV). I had to turn away from those things that I was substituting for God's Truth and allowing to be my master. Then, in order to have God be the only master of my life, I meditated daily on His Word so I could learn the Truth about beauty, my body, and good health. Because when you know the Truth, it will set you free from whatever bondage has enslaved you (John 8:32, NIV).

Taking It to Heart

1. What idol have you manufactured?

2. What have you allowed into your mind through your eyes and ears that has helped you manufacture your false idol?

3. How has that idol become your master?

Heavenly Father and Daughter Time

First, repent of replacing God with a manufactured idol. Then spend time in His Word, seeking His Truth that tears down that idol. Speak His Truth and meditate on His Truth so that you may be free from the bondage of a worthless idol.

Temple Tip for the Day

For the next 3 days, fast from those things that have contributed to building your false idol, such as beauty and gossip magazines, TV, and Internet feeds. ≈

Day 24

Uncompromising in the Face of Temptation

When you hear the word *compromise,* what pops into your head? For me, compromise is when I decide to go against what I know is the right thing to do. It can also be giving in to distractions and difficulties that test my character and convictions. No matter what your answer may be, there is one thing that all compromise has in common: it is preceded by temptation.

I am sure that by now many of you have been tempted not to stay committed to the fasting plan or the exercise plan or both. If you haven't been tempted I am happy for you. However, I find that I am continually tempted to put something into my mouth that I know will not produce good health in me, and I am often tempted to skip my exercise for the day. But as soon as I waver from my conviction to eat and exercise for good health, I feel guilty and start to beat myself up over my choice to compromise. So why do I compromise and why am I tempted?

I compromise because I am weak and I am tempted because I am enticed by own desires.

> *"Keep watch and pray, so that you will not give in to temptation. For the spirit is willing, but the body is weak!"*
>
> *Matthew 26:41 (NLT)*

> *Temptation comes from our own desires, which entice us and drag us away.*
>
> *James 1:14 (NLT)*

In Matthew 26:41, Jesus speaks to his disciples as they keep falling asleep in the Garden of Gethsemane right before His arrest and crucifixion. He had asked them to keep watch, but they gave in to their desire for rest and went to sleep. Their temptation was to sleep and in their weakness they were vulnerable to compromise. And that is where temptation will hit us: wherever we feel vulnerable. In our vulnerability we become weak toward what our flesh desires, and in our weakness we are tempted to compromise. But God does not abandon us when we are tempted; in fact, He becomes our strength to resist the temptation to compromise.

> *The temptations in your life are no different from what others experience. And God is faithful. He will not allow the temptation to be more than you can stand. When you are tempted, he will show a way out so that you can endure.*
>
> *1 Corinthians 10:13 (NLT)*

God reminds us that the temptations we face are not uncommon; others have been tempted in the same way. He tells us to trust Him because He will keep the temptation from becoming too strong and will show us a way out so we don't compromise. So how is that possible? In our weakness, He is strong (2 Corinthians 12:9). We cannot handle temptation on our own. We need to watch and pray—meaning we need to be aware that we will be tempted, and when temptation arises our first reaction should be to turn to Him, to call on His name and allow Him to give us the strength to walk away from the temptation.

OK, so sometimes we don't take the way out of the temptation and we compromise, for example, I eat a cupcake when I am on the fast. Now what? Of course I start to feel guilty and regret making that choice, and it is very easy to beat myself up over it. But 2 Corinthians 7:10 tells us that our regret can drive us to God's grace, forgiveness, and freedom, or we can allow it to push us away from God, which will only lead to guilt and condemnation. I'm not sure if eating that cupcake while committed to the fast qualifies as a sin for which I need forgiveness, but I do know that I want the freedom from guilt and regret that I feel from compromising, so I will seek God's grace.

Day 24 ~ Uncompromising

God warns us that we are vulnerable to temptation, but if we stop and pray He will show us how to resist and stand firm in our convictions. But He also tells us that if we choose to compromise, His grace is available to those who seek it.

Taking It to Heart

1. What is your greatest temptation to break the fast?

2. Why are you tempted by this?

3. What way has God revealed to you to get out of that temptation?

4. On a scale of 1 to 7 (with 1 being least and 7 being most), how willing are you to take that way out when faced with the temptation to compromise your commitment?

5. If your willingness is not a 7, what will it take to make it a 7?

Heavenly Father and Daughter Time

If you have compromised your commitment to this fast, offer your confession to the Lord and receive His grace. Pray to receive God's strength to take the way out of temptation that He has offered to you.

Temple Tip for the Day

When faced with the temptation to compromise your fast, stop and pray. Remember that through God you are strong enough to resist the temptation. And remember, nothing tastes as good as being healthy feels. ≈

Day 25

Planning for Profit

In the 1980s there was a popular television show called *The A Team*. One of the characters always came up with these unorthodox but effective plans for helping people. And at the end of every show he said, "I love it when a plan comes together." I can totally relate to that. I am a planner and I love when all my efforts come together beautifully, especially when it comes to our annual Christmas party. My husband and I spend months getting ready for this two-day event. We design and mail out invitations, and put a decorated tree and trimmings in every room in our house (which comes to a total of 13 trees), not to mention the light display outside. I take time to plan a diverse menu and prepare the food while my mother and mother-in-law bake dozens of cookies. We invite those who attend to bring an item to donate to our local crisis pregnancy center. Each year we welcome more than a hundred people into our home, and we have a fantastic time and accumulate an abundance for our local charity. At the end of that event we are extremely thankful for our guests' generosity, we feel blessed to be surrounded by so many wonderful people, and we can say we loved the time it took because our plan came together. I can't speak for the character from the TV show, but the reason I love it when plans work is because you can see the benefits were great both to the planner and to the people who were a part of the event.

Planning comes so naturally to me that sometimes I forget to include the Master Planner in my process—meaning that I often make my plans and then turn to God (if I even remember to turn to Him at all) and ask Him to bless them and make everything go smoothly. I can also at times exclude God from what I consider everyday tasks that take a little planning, such as planning my meals and snacks. I can honestly say that when I started this journey to better health I would plan my meals by consulting recipes and websites, but not once did I stop and ask God His thoughts on planning meals for the week.

I know there are great benefits to planning meals, such as managing your time better and making meal preparation easier. Planning ahead also helps you to avoid unhealthy choices, eliminates stress from having to make last-minute decisions about what to make for dinner, helps you to save time and money, makes grocery shopping easier, enables you to enjoy variety, and helps you to maintain a healthy, balanced diet. So I could only imagine the greater benefits that would come if I included, consulted, and committed my meal planning to the Lord.

The plans of the diligent lead to profit, as surely as haste leads to poverty.

Proverbs 21:5 (NIV)

I know that for some of us, meal planning can seem like a mundane task, but when patiently and diligently carried out it is a great accomplishment. Diligence is doing something with constant and persevering attention, and this does not come naturally to most people. It is a result of allowing God to build His character in us. Staying diligent in our task of meal planning can lead to success and be a positive tool in reaching our goals. However, we are often tempted to look for easy and quick ways to plan our meals, and that can lead to poor results and become a stumbling block to reaching our goals.

Plans fail for lack of counsel, but with many advisers they succeed.

Proverbs 15:22 (NIV)

When we lock our minds into one way of doing or thinking about things, we just might miss the right road because we have closed our minds to any new options. We need the help of those we know have experienced success in planning healthy meals because they can help us to enlarge our vision and broaden our perspective. Be open to new ideas and willing to weigh suggestions prayerfully. Our plans will become stronger and be more likely to succeed if we seek good counsel.

Commit to the Lord whatever you do, and your plans will succeed.

Proverbs 16:3 (NIV)

There are different ways that we can fail to commit whatever we do to the Lord. Sometimes we say we are doing it for the Lord but in reality we are doing it for ourselves. Other times we give God temporary or limited control of our plans, only to take the control back when things stop going the way we expected. And still other times we commit our plan fully to God but put forth no effort ourselves, and then we wonder why our plan failed. There is a balance between trusting God as if everything depended on Him while working as if everything depended on us.

If we diligently plan our meals, consult God first and then others who have set good examples, fully commit our plan to the Lord, and actively carry out the plan, our benefit will be success—the kind of success that has deepened our relationship with the Lord by depending on His guidance and trusting in His heart.

Taking It to Heart

1. How diligent are you in planning your meals and snacks?

2. Is your current commitment to meal planning creating profit or poverty? Explain.

3. How have you failed to commit your meal planning to the Lord?

4. How will you find balance between trusting God as if everything depended on Him while working as if everything depended on you?

Heavenly Father and Daughter Time

Before you plan your meals this week, ask your Heavenly Father to guide your decisions, then trust His ways as you follow His plan.

Temple Tip for the Day

When you find a recipe you like, keep it in a separate collection marked Blue Ribbon Recipes, or make a list of those recipes and where to find them as a quick go-to when planning your meals and snacks. ≈

Day 26

Two Lies We Believe About Time and Priorities: Lie #1

Time: Many of us, when we hear the word *time*, think, "I don't have enough of it" or "I don't use it wisely" or "It seems to pass so quickly."

Priorities: Priorities are those things that are of high importance and need attention first.

So, why are these two words important? Because we usually fill our *time* with what we consider to be our *priorities*, which is a very good thought, but then why do so many of us believe or feel that we are too busy or don't have enough time to get everything done, or that we've just got too much going on? We are overwhelmed by how much we have to do, bombarded by all the priorities that need our attention, and distressed by how little time we have to do them. All of this results in our living frazzled, discouraged lives, and that is what the enemy wants for us—a chaotic, busy life that distracts us from what God wants us to be doing.

The first lie about time and priorities that we have accepted is that we don't have enough time to do everything we are supposed to do. But the fact is that no person who has ever lived or who is living now has ever had more than 24 hours in a day, 168 hours in a week, and 52 weeks in a year. Jesus was given only a few short years on earth to accomplish the plan of redemption, and that was a task with a long to-do list. Yet in John 17:4 Jesus is able to say to

Day 26 ~ Lie #1 About Time and Priorities

His Father, "I have glorified thee on earth: I have finished the work which thou gavest me to do" (KJV).

And here is where we find the Truth that sets us free from the bondage of busyness and feeling like we don't have enough time to accomplish our to-do list. You see, Jesus didn't finish everything that the disciples asked Him to do or all that the multitudes of people wanted Him to do, but He finished the work that God gave Him to do. And just like Jesus, all we have to do is the work that God is asking us to do. Our freedom comes when we begin to accept that there is enough time for us to complete what God is asking us to do—today, this week, and in this lifetime.

Our bondage to busyness or feeling like we don't have enough time comes when we place tasks on our agenda without consulting God about whether He is even asking us to do those things. Or we ask God what He wants us to do with our day and then never slow down to hear the answer. Or maybe we let our perceived obligations dictate our schedules. Or maybe we just make our list and never talk to our Father about it other then when we get frustrated or discouraged or feel overwhelmed and need Him to rescue us from our busy day. And that is what happens when we attempt to take on responsibilities that are not on His agenda for us: we grow frustrated. When we let others dictate or determine our priorities, we end up overextended, overwhelmed, unfocused, and feeling like we haven't accomplished anything, rather than enjoying the peaceful, well-ordered life that God intended for us to have.

Imagine for a moment that you did not set your agenda for the day at all! Imagine that before you put pen to paper to make your to-do list you stopped, asked your Heavenly Father to show you the work He wanted you to do today, then waited and listened for His reply. Imagine that you let God dictate your priorities today. After all, He is the One who knows you best. He is the One who has designed your life with a purpose.

> *"For I know the plans I have for you," declares the* LORD, *"plans to prosper you and not to harm you, plans to give you hope and a future."*
>
> *Jeremiah 29:11 (NIV)*

Faith and Fitness for Life

God knows the plan He has for your life. He already knows what He desires for your day, week, and life. His plan brings hope and causes us to thrive. He wants to share that plan with us, but we have to be willing to trust His ways and be obedient to His plan.

> *Trust in the LORD with all your heart and lean not on your own understanding; in all your ways submit to him, and he will make your paths straight.*
>
> *Proverbs 3:5–6 (NIV)*

The more time we spend with God, the more we trust Him. The more we trust the Lord, the more we rely on His wisdom and not on our own. The more we rely on His wisdom, the more we are willing to consult Him in all that we do. And the more we consult Him in all our ways, the more we see the plan that He has designed for us. When we see His plan for our day, we can choose to follow His design. The more we follow His design for our day, the more we accept that there is enough time in our day to accomplish the to-do list that God has prepared for us, and we are freed from the lie.

Taking It to Heart

1. Who or what is influencing the priorities on your to-do list?

2. What would it look like to consult God before making your to-do list for the day?

3. How would it feel to be able to accomplish all that God has placed on your to-do list?

4. What would it get you to allow God to make your to-do list?

5. What next step could you take toward allowing God to share His plan for your day, week, and/or life?

6. When will you take that step?

7. What might stop you from taking that step?

8. How could you minimize that interference?

Heavenly Father and Daughter Time

Consult your Heavenly Father before making your plans today. Spend time listening for His voice to show you the path for your day.

Temple Tip for the Day

Don't confuse thirst with hunger. Drink a glass of water when you feel hungry before eating a snack to see if that is what you are really craving. ≈

Day 27

Two Lies We Believe About Time and Priorities: Lie #2

There is another lie about our time and priorities that we women have accepted and that is, "I can do it all." We believe that we should be able to be an ideal mother and wife, keep the house clean and organized, prepare healthy meals, be active in church life and in the kids' schools and sports, stay physically fit, keep up with current events, keep the budget in order, and have a job outside the home (feel free to add to the list). But the truth is, no woman can wear all of these hats effectively. Sooner or later something or someone will suffer.

If we believe that we are able to juggle all those roles, we will find ourselves exhausted and overwhelmed by all the demands on our time. And these feelings are warning signs telling us that we are buying into the lie that we can do it all. But God didn't design us to "do it all." In fact, He designed us to do only those things that He planned for us a long time ago.

For we are God's masterpiece. He has created us anew in Christ Jesus, so we can do the good things he planned for us long ago.

Ephesians 2:10 (NLT)

Masterpiece is defined as the most outstanding piece of creative work of a craftsman or artist. *You* are God's most outstanding piece of art. He has created you like no other, not just in the way you look but for what He has designed you to do. Because He created the masterpiece of you, He already knows the tasks your day, week, and life will hold. It is we who need to seek God's priorities, the good things He has planned for us to do.

> *However, I consider my life worth nothing to me, if only I may finish the race and complete the task the Lord Jesus has given me.*
>
> *Acts 20:24 (NIV)*

Paul thought his life was worth nothing unless he completed the task that Jesus had given him. He wasn't concerned with being able to do it all or with doing the same tasks that someone else had been given; he concerned himself only with finishing the tasks that Jesus have given Him to complete. So, not only do we want to take the time to find out what tasks God is asking us to complete, but we also want to remember that our to-do list for today or for life is not the same as anyone else's. What God is asking you to do is exclusive to you. That's what a masterpiece is: a one-of-a-kind.

Taking It to Heart

1. How has the lie that "I can do it all" been manifested in how you spend your time?

Day 27 ~ Lie #2 About Time and Priorities

2. What has been the result of believing you can do it all?

3. How would your schedule be different if you didn't feel you needed to do it all?

4. What one word describes how you feel knowing that God created you as a masterpiece?

5. How will knowing that God created you with unique tasks in mind change the way you plan your time and choose your priorities?

Heavenly Father and Daughter Time

Ask your Heavenly Father to reveal your unique tasks for the day. Thank and praise Him for the beautiful work of art He created in you.

Temple Tip for the Day

Sodium makes us bloated. Potassium helps reduce water retention. Try to choose foods low in sodium or high in potassium to help lessen water retention. ≈

Day 28

Validated Through Approval

As far back as I can remember I have wanted to be a musician. I have been playing piano and singing since I was 5 years old. I love music so much that I majored in voice and minored in piano at college. For 25 years music has been my career in one form or another. I have been an elementary school music teacher, director of musicals in kids' community theaters, private piano and vocal instructor, recording and touring artist, choral conductor, worship leader, and worship leader trainer. Through the years I have been privileged to work with many talented adults and kids—and you have probably never heard of any of them. But although they are not famous and their names are not well-known, they are individuals with incredible talent unique to themselves.

Currently the majority of my teaching is with vocal students. When I have a new student I always start by asking, what the goal is for taking lessons and what the student dreams of doing with his or her talent. Usually the response is, "I want to get better at singing" and to sing on Broadway or be the next rock star. I love that my students want to master their talent, and I even love that they are dreaming big. However, it breaks my heart when my students believe that the only way they can feel good about their talent and claim success is if they become famous, and that if they don't become famous or recognized for their ability, their talent isn't good enough. Of course I reassure them that they don't need fame in order to be a successful musician; many musicians have a successful career in music and no one knows their name except their family and friends.

Maybe the idea of young people believing that only fame means success and that they need fame in order to feel good about themselves and their talent breaks your heart as well. But isn't that what we do too? Don't we measure our success on the basis of whether we are approved of and validated as good enough? And let's face it: we all like the idea of being approved of and validated as important. But the problem lies in seeking that approval and validation from a source other than God.

> *Am I now trying to win the approval of men, or of God? Or am I trying to please men? If I were still trying to please men, I would not be a servant of Christ.*
> Galatians 1:10 (NIV)

If we are seeking to be approved of and accepted by people, we have placed the value of their opinion of us above being a servant of Christ. When we value man's opinion over God's, we say and do things in an effort to please people so that they will accept us. We begin to find our sense of value and worth from what others think of us instead of from our identity in Christ. Seeking their approval will begin to dictate our behavior. We will do things to gain people's approval or to get a compliment, which feels good for a moment but then that feeling wears off and we are left with the same feelings we started with—a sense of lacking worth and value, and an insecurity about who we are. If we want a permanent sense of value, worth, and security, we must begin seeking God's approval and not people's.

> *Our purpose is to please God, not people. He alone examines the motives of our hearts.*
> 1 Thessalonians 2:4 (NLT)

> *"But seek first His Kingdom and His righteousness, and all these things will be given to you as well."*
> Matthew 6:33 (NIV)

To seek first His Kingdom and righteousness means that we actively choose to give Him first place in every area of our lives, including the need to feel approved of and validated. When we seek His righteousness, we find our true value, worth, and identity.

Day 28 ~ Validated Through Approval

When we understand who we are in Christ, we understand that through His death and resurrection we have been accepted and approved of as children of God. And as children of God our purpose is to walk in obedience to what He is calling us to do, which is pleasing to Him. We do this not out of obligation but out of a heart motive of gratitude and love for what He has done for us.

> *Whatever you do, work at it with all your heart, as working for the Lord, not for men, since you know that you will receive an inheritance from the Lord as a reward. It is the Lord Christ you are serving.*
>
> *Colossians 3:23–24 (NIV)*

Working for the approval and validation of men will give us a temporary inheritance of worth and value that will quickly fade. But when we serve the Lord with all our heart, doing what is pleasing to Him, we will be blessed to hear Him say, "Well done, my good and faithful servant"—a reward that is eternal.

Taking It to Heart

1. In what or whom do you seek your worth and value?

2. Do you need compliments from people to validate your worth or to know that you are good enough?

3. How do your actions show that you are seeking God's approval and not man's?

Heavenly Father and Daughter Time

Seek first God's Kingdom and His righteousness in all that you do. Ask Him to search your heart and reveal your true heart motive in seeking approval and validation. Journal about what God reveals to you.

Temple Tip for the Day

Cut back on your carbohydrate intake. Eat only lean protein and veggies for dinner. ≈

Day 29

Unwrapping Your Gift and Giving It Away

Every Christian has been given a gift. It is much like a birthday gift: you have done nothing to earn it. When you were saved it was freely given to you by the Holy Spirit, who came to live within you.

> *It is the one and only Spirit who distributes all these gifts. He alone decides which gift each person should have.*
>
> 1 Corinthians 12:11 (NLT)

And just as the gift giver expects us to do with a birthday gift, God expects us to unwrap the gift He has given and use it—not for ourselves but to serve others and build up the body of Christ.

> *Each one should use whatever gift he has received to serve others, faithfully administering God's grace in its various forms.*
>
> 1 Peter 4:10 (NIV)

Why would God give us a gift and then expect us to give it away to others by serving them? The answer is simple: "For even the Son of Man came not to be served but to serve others and to give his life as a ransom for many" Matthew 20:28, NIV). As Christians we are to imitate the life of Christ, and this scripture clearly explains that God sent His Son to humbly serve others, not use His power and glory to promote Himself. And that is what He expects of us as well: to humbly serve others with the gifts He has given us, not use them to promote ourselves.

To be humble means to be not proud or arrogant. Philippians 2:3–4 says, "Don't be selfish; don't try to impress others. Be humble, thinking of others as better than yourselves. Don't look out only for your own interests, but take an interest in others, too" (NLT). This means not that we put ourselves down but rather that we have the same attitude as Christ. Christ's attitude of humility in serving was sacrificial; He laid aside selfish ambition and treated others with respect and common courtesy. I don't know about all of you but for me pride comes more naturally than humility, and for that reason humility is a character trait we must choose to nurture. By fostering an attitude of gratefulness, we can begin to nurture an attitude of humility. "But be sure to fear the LORD and serve him faithfully with all your heart; consider what great things he has done for you" (1 Samuel 12:24, NLT). Reflecting on the many great things that God has done for us strengthens our faith and focuses our motives on God and not on our own gain.

Being a servant means being a person in service to another. When we give Jesus lordship over our lives, we become servants of the King. If we are in service to our King, we have agreed to use our gifts, talents, and time to do that to which He has called us. Romans 12:4–8 and Ephesians 4:11–12 teach us that all gifts and abilities come from God and that not all of us have the same gift but *all* gifts are valuable in the building of the body of Christ. Knowing who we are and what gifts and abilities God has blessed us with allows us to contribute effectively to the building of God's Kingdom.

Often we think we don't have anything to contribute or maybe we covet others' gifts. But you can see in these scriptures that each of us and our gifts, no matter what they are, are needed for the Body of Christ to thrive. And Ephesians 2:10 tells us that we are *all* created to do the good works that God prepared in advance for us to do.

If we are going to complete the good works that God has prepared for us to do, we must first unwrap and discover the gifts that the Holy Spirit has given us, and then we must give them away by using them in humble service to others.

Day 29 ~ Unwrapping Your Gift

Taking It to Heart

1. Take time to discover the gifts and abilities you have been given. Ask God to reveal them to you. You may also take a spiritual gift test (I recommend an online version at www.uniquelyyou.com) and/or ask people you know and trust what they see you are good at.

2. What are you passionate about? What excites you?

3. How can you combine your passion with your gifts and abilities?

4. In what way does using your gifts and abilities build up the Body of Christ? Remember that *all* functions are necessary in the building up of the Body of Christ.

Heavenly Father and Daughter Time

Spend time recalling all of the great things that your Heavenly Father has done for you. Start a thankfulness journal in which to record the great things He has done for you in the past and the great things he does for you on each day going forward. Then take time to reflect on these things so that you can begin to nurture your humble servant's heart.

Temple Tip for the Day

Take time today to do something nice for someone else. Write a note of encouragement, help someone organize a closet—be creative here! Remember, the idea is to serve another humbly in an effort to build them up. ≈

Day 30

Comparing Yourself to Others

Have you ever compared yourself to others? Have you ever thought your gifts were not as important as another's or envied someone else's gifts? Or maybe you've thought you have nothing to offer, or that what you have to offer is more important than what someone else is giving? If you answered yes to any of these questions, you are comparing yourself to others.

Comparing comes almost as naturally as breathing. We often do it without even thinking. But when we compare, we are either putting ourselves down or judging others and seeing ourselves as better than them. One thought makes us feel bad and the other makes us feel superior. Either way we are more focused on others and what they are doing than on what God is asking us to do with what we have been given.

> *Make a careful exploration of who you are and the work you have been given, and then sink yourself into that. Don't be impressed with yourself. Don't compare yourself with others. Each of you must take responsibility for doing the creative best you can with your own life.*
>
> Galatians 6:4–5 (MSG)

Clearly God's Word is telling us not to compare ourselves to others and not to think too highly of ourselves. But why would God instruct us not to compare ourselves to others? I believe He wants to warn us of the dangers of comparing. In the scripture just quoted, Paul begins by encouraging us to "make a careful exploration" of who we are and what we have been asked to do. He wants us to discover our identity and what God's call is for us. Who we are is not defined by our physical appearance, family, friends, church membership, place of residence, career, or past. Who we are is defined by the Word of God. And His Word says we are His daughters, one-of-a-kind creations with a combination of gifts, talents, and abilities that no one else possesses. And God has given each of us a unique function that only we can fulfill.

Notice that Paul instructs us to make a "careful" exploration. This is because when we begin to consider our potential there is danger that we will compare ourselves to others. We may begin to think too highly of ourselves, that we are better than others. But Galations 6:4–5 also says "Don't be impressed with yourself." When we think too highly of ourselves not only are we looking down on and thinking less of others, but we also often get ideas about our life that are unrealistic and totally out of line with how God has made us. On the other end of the comparison spectrum, we can also think too little of ourselves. Further in the same scripture Paul says, "But try to have a sane estimate of your capabilities by the light of the faith that God has given to you all," which means that underestimating our potential stops us from using the gifts and talents that God has given us, and we lose the motivation to take our own potential seriously. In a way, when we do that we are saying that what God has given us or who God has created us to be isn't good enough.

Either way in which we compare ourselves to others has the same result: we fail to take responsibility for doing our best with the gifts, talents, and abilities that God has given us to complete the work to which He has called us. That is why Paul, in Galatians 6, also encourages us to take the next step when we begin to understand our gifts, talents, and abilities: "sink yourself into that." Embrace how God has gifted you and seek His guidance on what to do with it. Psalm 139:16 (NIV) says, "All the days ordained for me were written in your book before one of them came to be." Here God is telling us that He's got us! He has placed on our lives an honorable gift and has planned ways that we can use it for His Kingdom. Sinking in to who we are and into the work God has called us to do means that we are enveloped by our identity in Christ and the work He wants us to do in a way that blocks out all

Day 30 ~ Comparing Yourself to Others

desire to compare ourselves to others. We see ourselves as God sees us: unique, wonderful, talented, and gifted!

Taking It to Heart

1. How have you compared yourself to others during this time of fasting?

2. Describe other ways that you compare yourself to others?

3. How does that comparing make you feel?

4. How has that comparing affected your motivation to stay focused on your goals during this time of fasting? How has comparing affected your calling from God?

5. What step(s) can you take to understand who you are in Christ and the work He has called you to complete?

6. When will you take that step?

7. How will you be held accountable in taking that step?

Heavenly Father and Daughter Time

Grab a pen and paper. Get comfortable. Invite your Heavenly Father to be with you in this time and ask Him this question: "God, when you look at me, what do you see?" It might take a few minutes to quiet your mind and that is OK. If distractions creep in just let them pass through your mind and focus on the question again. Write down any words or images that God gives you during this time.

Temple Tip for the Day

Try replacing one meal with a healthy, balanced smoothie. You'll enjoy the change, and the fewer calories! ≈

Day 31

Give It a Rest!

I am so proud of my stepdaughter and how hard she works. For 4 years she worked in a nursing home as a homemaker, and she recently graduated from training and received her license to be a CNA (Certified Nursing Assistant). Now she is working as a CNA at a new nursing home while taking extra shifts at her previous nursing home. The child is not afraid to work. Of course as her parents we get concerned about the number of hours she is working and about how tired she sometimes looks from her long days. We have encouraged her to slow down and consider focusing on her CNA work so she gets proper rest and doesn't wear herself out. And her response to us has been, "I can rest when I'm dead."

Now, I don't know about you but in our neck of the woods that statement is used fairly commonly when a person is working nonstop and lacking proper rest. We use it as an excuse for our devotion to busyness. But honestly the statement makes no sense to me. I can rest when I'm dead? What's the point of resting when I'm dead? I think by then it will be too late for rest—you know what I mean? And besides, when I'm dead I'll be in heaven with the saints who have gone before me, having a fabulous time worshiping God and seeing Jesus face to face. Why would I take a nap then? But in all seriousness, we do need rest.

Think for a moment about what you are like when you haven't gotten enough rest. I become cranky and impatient and have trouble focusing. I feel weary and have no energy to do anything, even the things I like to do. Is any of this sounding familiar to you? Not only does sleep deprivation affect our moods and concentration levels but it also can alter the level of our body's hormones that regulate hunger, causing an increase in appetite, and can affect the

Day 31 ~ Give It a Rest!

way our bodies process and store carbohydrates giving us the potential for weight gain. Have you ever noticed what you do during the day when you are feeling tired? I would usually reach for a cup of coffee or something to eat. But what I really needed was proper rest.

From the beginning God has shown us that we need rest. Look at the story of creation (Genesis 1 and 2). God spoke light and darkness into existence and called the light day and the darkness night, "and there was an evening, and there was a morning." That statement is heard on each day of creation. I think God is trying to tell us something here. He has given us time to rest (evening) and time to work (morning). Through His gifts of evening and morning, God is showing us that our bodies need proper rest.

And God has given us another gift of rest and that is the gift of the Sabbath.

> *By the seventh day God had finished the work he had been doing; so on the seventh day He rested from all His work. And God blessed the seventh day and made it holy, because on it He rested from all the work of creating that He had done.*
>
> *Genesis 2:2–3 (NIV)*

God took a day to rest from all the work He had done. He blessed it and set it apart for holy use. It seems like there is always something to be done, and we can make excuses for working constantly. But if God took time to rest from His work, then we shouldn't be surprised that He asks the same of us. (Exodus 20:1–7). God gave us the gift of the Sabbath to serve us (Mark 2:27) because He knew we would need a day to rest from our busy schedules on the other days and to renew our physical strength. But rest is also needed so that we may know peace.

> *Then Jesus said, "Come to me, all of you who are weary and carry heavy burdens, and I will give you rest."*
>
> *Matthew 11:28 (NLT)*

Jesus invites us to come to Him, to entrust our worries and responsibilities to Him, and to rest. He wants to give us rest, the kind of rest that allows us to know peace, not just the absence of work. But resting means we must trust that God will take care of things for us. We must trust that our world will not stop functioning if we rest, because we are not the ones making if function in the first place. When it comes to resting from a busy schedule, Jesus has set the example for us to follow:

Then Jesus said, "Let's go off by ourselves to a quiet place and rest awhile." He said this because there were so many people coming and going that Jesus and his apostles didn't even have time to eat.

Mark 6:31 (NLT)

Jesus didn't wait for an open spot in His schedule to slow down and rest. He rested in the midst of being in demand. He did this because He understands that if we want to be effective in our work, our bodies and minds need quiet and rest so that we will be strengthened and have good health. He did this because He understood that we all need to withdraw from our busy schedules to find the peace that comes from being still and hearing the voice of God. It is easy for us to say that we can't stop and rest until we are finished with such-and-such or until we are done with our to-do lists. But Jesus demonstrated that rest is a choice. We can choose either to rest in order to gain strength and peace or we can choose to keep our schedules so filled that we gain stress and anxiety and become worn out and ineffective.

Taking It to Heart

1. Is your current schedule bringing you strength and peace or is it wearing you out?

Day 31 ~ Give It a Rest!

2. What would it look like to have a Sabbath?

3. What would you gain by taking the gift of a Sabbath?

4. What would it look like to have a schedule that reflects Jesus's example?

5. What would you gain by adjusting your schedule to imitate Jesus, who took time to withdraw and be still in order to find peace and relief?

6. What step(s) could you take to follow Jesus's example and gain the peace and relief of the Sabbath?

Heavenly Father and Daughter Time

In your time today with your Heavenly Father just be still and quiet and know that He is your God.

Temple Tip for the Day

Get proper sleep! For the next week make room in your schedule for a 20-minute nap during the day. You don't need to sleep; just be still and for 20 minutes hand everything over to God. ≈

Day 32

Listen When Your Body Is Speaking

If anyone destroys God's temple, God will destroy him; for God's temple is sacred, and you are that temple.

1 Corinthians 3:17 (NIV)

God has designed our bodies to talk to us. For example, do you ever feel like you don't have enough physical energy to get through the day? I am sure most of us have felt this way at times. So what do we do? If you are like I was, you reach for a cup of coffee or a sugary treat as a pick-me-up. When I did this, it gave me a temporary lift in energy but I would soon find myself back to feeling like I had no energy. So what did I do? I'd have another cup of coffee. The cycle would continue until I got a headache and indigestion from all the coffee I was drinking, and I felt even more exhausted because of the energy ups and downs I had put my body through. My body was telling me it needed energy, but I was responding in a way that was destroying the temple!

We would never dream of walking into our church building with a bag of smelly trash and dumping it all over the floor, yet that is exactly what we are doing when we use a substance to silence our body's voice that is telling us something is wrong. When I was experiencing a lack of energy, it was because I wasn't getting enough rest. I didn't wake up feeling exhausted, but I also didn't wake up feeling refreshed.

God placed a warning system inside our bodies to let us know when we are on the path to temple destruction. The system starts with little signals like fatigue or maybe headaches or stomach problems or physical pain. When we ignore these little signals, our body responds with a louder signal, such as the onset of sickness or complete exhaustion. And if we still insist on ignoring the warning signs, our bodies eventually give up and break down.

Is your body giving you warning signs? Ask yourself these questions:

1. How do you feel after you eat a meal or snack?
2. Do you have trouble sleeping?
3. Do you get frequent headaches?
4. Are your ears and throat always itchy?
5. Do you suffer from chapped lips?
6. Are you continually constipated or having other digestive problems?
7. Do you wake up feeling refreshed or exhausted?
8. Do you frequently get a cold?
9. Do you have enough energy to make it through the day?
10. Do you suffer from constant bloating, gas, or both?

These are just a few of the signs that can tell us that something is wrong. It is not normal to encounter these symptoms frequently. The sad part is that some of us don't take these warning signs seriously, or we just resign ourselves to the fact that this is just how we are always going to feel and that we just have to put up with our discomfort.

But God desires good health for us, meaning daily exercise, good nutrition, and adequate rest, and because He wants us to have good health He designed our bodies to talk to us and let us know when something is wrong. And he has shown us how to respond to those signs—not to take a shortcut and pop a pill for temporary relief, but to treat our body as the sacred temple it is. We must do our part and eat nourishing food, exercise to strengthen our bodies, and get adequate rest. How can God give us the blessing of good health if we continue to trash our temple?

Day 32 ~ When Your Body Is Speaking

Taking It to Heart

1. Answer the questions about warning signs in today's devotion.

2. What is your body telling you through the questions you answered yes to?

3. What step or steps can you take to stop trashing your temple?

4. When will you take those steps?

5. What might stop you from taking those steps?

6. How can you minimize that interference?*

Heavenly Father and Daughter Time

Pray that your Heavenly Father will help you to stay committed to the steps you are taking to stop trashing your temple, and be obedient to what He is revealing to you through your body.

Temple Tip for the Day

Remember to eat as many whole foods as you can, keeping them as raw as possible. Raw foods help to burn fat and contain many nutrients. ≈

---

* If your symptoms persist, please consult your family doctor.

Day 33

Dream Big

My dad and I are often accused of having some pretty crazy dreams. To most people they make no sense whatsoever, but those dreams excite us and dare us to do and be more. Our imaginations run wild with possibilities and plans. But most of those crazy dreams we have never come to fruition. Why? Well, just because we have a dream does not mean we are meant to act on it. In fact, Andy Stanley, in his book *Visioneering*, encourages us to wait. But while we wait we are to pray, and as we do so it will become clear if our dream is God-ordained, we will give God time to prepare us to act, and we will give Him time to make the way clear. But there are other reasons we often don't act on a crazy dream, even when it is from God. One reason is that the dream seems so big we think there is no way we can achieve it, so we don't even try. Another reason is that we belittle the dream by thinking it seems insignificant, so we dismiss it's value and don't follow through.

Let's begin to address these reasons by understanding that *all* of us have been called by our Heavenly Father. The same God who saved us also gave us a holy calling before time began. And just as we did nothing to earn our salvation, we also have done nothing to earn the call He has placed on our life.

> *God, who saved us and called us to a holy calling, not because of our works but because of his own purpose and grace, which he gave us in Christ Jesus before the ages began.*
>
> 2 Timothy 1:9 (ESV)

But God does not call us and then abandon us to figure things out on our own. He equips us with what we need to do His will. He provides the skills, abilities, and resources, and the how.

> *May He equip you with all you need for doing His will. May He produce in you, through the power of Jesus Christ, every good thing that is pleasing to Him. All glory to Him forever and ever! Amen.*
>
> *Hebrews 13:21 (NLT)*

Clearly we can see that *all* have been called and that God will equip us for that calling. So why do we then believe that the dream, the calling, is so big that we can't fulfill it, or why do we think our dream is not important? We believe these things because we have bought into lies like "I have to rely on myself to achieve the dream" and "I am not valuable, so why would my calling be valuable?" And we compare our dream to those of others and in our eyes it seems little and insignificant. Regardless of the lie we believe, the result is the same: we are not living out the call on our life and therefore are not building up the body of Christ and bringing God glory.

If you believe that your dream is so big you can't do it, then you are right! *You* can't achieve the holy calling that God has placed on your life without God. He will equip you with everything you need to do His will.

> *For it is God who works in you to will and to act according to his good purpose.*
>
> *Philippians 2:13 (NIV)*

Again we see that it is God who is producing in us what we will need. The Lord Jesus Christ will guides us and shows us each step we should take (Isaiah 58:11), and He encourages us, telling us that we can do all things through His power (Philippians 4:13).

Day 33 ~ Dream Big

Just as our bodies have many parts and each part has a special function, so it is with Christ's body. We are many parts of one body, and we all belong to each other.
Romans 12:4–5 (NLT)

You and your calling, your dream, are valuable and significant. You and your God-given dream are a part of the body of Christ. Your dream has a special function that can be fulfilled only by you with the gifts and talents that God has given and equipped you with. No one's function is more important than another's; all parts belong to each other and all parts are needed to help each other as we build up the body of Christ.

God calls us and God equips us and God never leaves us alone on the journey. And because of these Truths our response should always be, "Here I am Lord, send me" (Isaiah 6:8).

Taking It to Heart

1. What crazy dream(s) have you had?

2. Were they God-ordained or just imagination run wild?

3. If they were God-ordained, did you follow through?

4. If yes, explain your experience. If not, what stopped you from following through?

5. How can you prevent that roadblock from happening again?

Heavenly Father and Daughter Time

Imagine God is handing you a big, beautiful box. The box is so enormous that you cannot hold it on your own. There has never been and never will be another box just like this one. And God says it belongs to you and only you. In it is God's dream for you. Open the box and allow God to reveal the dream inside, your holy calling. Journal about what is revealed. Invite your Heavenly Father to provide and equip you with all you will need to do His will.

Temple Tip for the Day

When you eat at a restaurant ask the server to hold the bread, chips and salsa, or other snack food that might come before the meal. If you are hungry you'll be tempted to eat that instead of or on top of your healthy menu choice. ≈

Day 34

W.A.I.T.

> They that wait upon the Lord shall renew their strength
> They will mount up with wings like eagles
> They will run and not grow weary
> They will walk and not faint
> Teach me Lord, teach me Lord to wait.
>
> *Words and Music by Stuart Hamblen,*
> *© 1953/1981 Hamblen Music Company*

Teach me Lord to wait. What a wonderful and challenging request. Isaiah 40:31 (NIV) says, "but those who hope in the Lord will renew their strength. They will soar on wings like eagles; they will run and not grow weary, they will walk and not faint."

Waiting does not mean we stop, stand still, and do nothing. Rather, to wait means to serve or attend to, to patiently anticipate (www.dictionary.com). But what are we waiting for, what are we patiently anticipating?

> *For this hope we are saved. But hope that is seen is no hope at all. Who hopes for what he already has? But if we hope for what we do not yet have, we wait for it patiently.*
> Romans 8:24–25 (NIV)

We are waiting patiently for Christ's return, but not by just sitting around idly, watching life go by. Waiting takes action. While we wait for Christ's return we are to be serving the living and true God. Hoping and waiting in the Lord renews our strength because it reminds us that we are not in this alone. We can expect that His promise of strength will help us to rise above life's distractions, doubts, and difficulties.

While I was in school earning my certification to be a Christian Life Coach, our instructor shared with us the acronym W.A.I.T., which means "Why am I talking?" She told us to use this acronym to remind ourselves that being a great coach means that 20 percent of the time we are talking and 80 percent of the time we are listening to our clients. As I was learning to be a great listener for my clients, I began to wonder if I was a great listener to God.

So often when I approach my quiet time with the Lord I have *my* list of intercessory prayer requests, *my* list of praise and thanksgiving, *my* list of what I need His help with, *my agenda*. Make no mistake: our Lord wants to hear all of these things from us. But *my* agenda is *not* what gives me renewed strength to rise above the troubles of this life. It is His presence with us and His Word to us that renews us daily. But we need to take action and wait, we need to take action and listen. If 80 percent of the time I am talking to God and 20 percent of the time I am listening, am I really receiving *all* that God wants to give to me? Imagine if we spoke only 20 percent of the time we spent with God and listened 80 percent of the time: how much more would we receive?

I have learned to wait while I coach in order to discover my client's agendas, dreams, plans, and obstacles. I believe that God too wants us to wait in Him so that He may reveal *His* agenda, dreams, and plans for us and prepare us for the obstacles that may lie ahead. If we never stop talking long enough to hear *all* that God has to say, we truly miss out on the abundant peace, hope, and strength that He promises to His children.

Spend time talking to your Heavenly Father and then wait; don't rush away so quickly. Allow His voice and His presence to renew your strength so that you may rise, like the eagles, above the troubles of this life. Allow the hope you find while you patiently anticipate His return renew your strength so that you may not grow weary while running or walking at the pace of the call He has placed on your life.

Taking It to Heart

1. On a scale of 1 to 7, with 7 being the best and 1 being the worst, how would you rate your listening skills?

2. When you spend time with the Lord, what percentage of that time are you talking? What percentage are you listening?

3. Describe what it would be like just to be still and actively listen for God's agenda, dreams, plans, and warnings about obstacles.

Day 34 ~ W.A.I.T.

4. What would you need to make that happen?

5. What is the next step you can take toward spending more time listening to God and less time talking to Him?

6. When will you take that next step?

7. How will you hold yourself accountable for that step?

8. What other resources might you need?

Heavenly Father and Daughter Time

Pray this prayer: Heavenly Father, thank you for giving me hope—a hope that gives me strength, a hope that gives me peace and a future. Lord, renew me with *your* strength so that I may not focus on my present circumstances but instead rise above as the overcomer you have created me to be. But most of all, Lord, teach me to wait *in* You. In Your Name I pray. Amen.

Temple Tip for the Day

Avoid eating while watching television or in a movie theater, while scrolling through Facebook or YouTube, and so on. These things are dining distractions and will cause you to eat more calories. ≈

Day 35

Love Expressed

Growing up I was very close to my Nannie; that's what we called my Grandmother. She was a beautiful, loving woman who cared for many children in her lifetime. In addition to raising her own four children, she also raised a niece, spent more than 40 years nurturing and raising countless foster children, and provided day care for dozens of children from her hometown—not to mention all the grandkids who would have sleepovers and hang out at her house when their parents were working. My mom shares a story about how once when she dropped my brother and me at Nannie's house she counted 22 children—foster children, day care children, and grandchildren—playing in the yard. I loved being there, not just because there were always kids to play with, but also because when you were there you felt loved. My Nannie expressed her love by playing with us when we were little. If she hadn't seen us for a few days she would pursue us by calling our parents and have them bring us over for a visit. And during my four years of college she took the time to write me a letter every week. Those are just a few ways she loved us. I could always count on my Nannie to say just the right thing to make me feel better when I was feeling down. She never gave up on me and always believed in me.

> *Love is patient and kind. Love is not jealous or boastful or proud or rude. It does not demand its own way. It is not irritable, and it keeps no record of being wronged. It does not rejoice about injustice but rejoices whenever the truth wins out. Love never gives up, never loses faith, is always hopeful, and endures through every circumstance.*
>
> *1 Corinthians 13:4–7 (NLT)*

The love that God defines is the kind that will encourage and build up the people we say we love or who say they love us (1 Thessalonians 5:11). It is sacrificial, forgiving, and generous. It is the same kind of love that God shows toward us (John 3:16, Romans 5:8). That's the kind of love my Nannie showed toward me.

But it is also the kind of love that does not come naturally to most people. It is easier for us to lose our cool with our spouse, or to be jealous of a friend, or to want things done our way. It has become acceptable that when things get tough we just end the relationship, or we store up old offenses to use against the person in an opportune moment. But that is not the kind of love that God wants for us or wants us to give to others.

On many occasions as I was growing up I heard the phrase "don't act so dumb" from different sources when I was not using common sense—and for a child that can happen quite often. Although those words were meant not to harm but to guide, my heart interpreted them as "Lisa, you are dumb." And that is what I grew up believing: that I was dumb. In my adult life, as I shared earlier, I dated a man who was verbally, emotionally, and physically abusive to me. His degrading words made me feel worthless even though he said he loved me; his hurtful words and fists did not feel loving. This is why in Ephesians and Romans Paul instructs us in how to express our love toward one another.

> *Don't use foul or abusive language. Let everything you say be good and helpful, so that your words will be an encouragement to those who hear them.*
>
> *Ephesians 4:9 (NLT)*

> *Therefore, let us stop passing judgment on one another. Instead, make up your mind not to put any stumbling block or obstacle in your brother's way.*
>
> *Romans 14:13 (NIV)*

We express love through actions and words. If the love we give and receive is motivated by the love that's described in 1 Corinthians 13, then the things we say and do should build up, encourage, strengthen, and minister grace toward us and those we love. But again, for most of us this does not come naturally. We have to intentionally choose words that are good and helpful so that the person receiving them will feel encouraged. And our actions speak just as loud as if not louder than our words. So we must also use God's wisdom in how we treat each other. If we don't, there is the potential for us to create a stumbling block or obstacle in the person's life. When our words and actions discourage and tear down, we create a hurt that causes a stumbling block, essentially hindering their spiritual growth and blocking their understanding of their value and worth. One stumbling block came as a result of believing the lie that I was dumb, which broke down my confidence. Another was the feelings of worthlessness that came from the abuse I experienced, which created in me disbelief that my life had any value.

Our words and actions have the power to bring life or death, encouragement or discouragement. When we talk to each other or about each other, we should strive to show the love that is described in 1 Corinthians 13; then we will bring life to others, by encouraging them and building them up in Christ. So, not only did my Nannie set an example for me of how to love, but she also taught me a precious Truth from scripture that still serves as a reminder to love others with my words and actions.

"So in everything, do to others what you would have them do to you."

Matthew 7:12 NIV

Taking It to Heart

1. In 1 Corinthians 13, which description of love do you find most challenging?

2. Why?

3. Describe how your words and actions have expressed or currently express love?

4. Describe how your words and actions have torn someone down or discouraged them?

Day 35 ~ Love Expressed

5. Describe how you felt when someone who loved you was discouraging or abusive with their words or actions?

6. How can that feeling motivate you in how you love others?

Heavenly Father and Daughter Time

Pray for guidance and wisdom as you mindfully choose actions and words that express the 1 Corinthians kind of love. If your words and actions have not been encouraging and have not built others up, ask your Heavenly Father for forgiveness, accept His mercy and grace, and begin anew by speaking and acting mindfully according to the instructions in scripture.

Temple Tip for the Day

Take time to savor your food. It makes eating more enjoyable and helps you to control your appetite. If you eat too quickly you may not sense when you are full and satisfied. Try putting your fork down between bites and chewing more slowly. ≈

Day 36

Made in the Image of God

There I was, standing in front of the mirror. For 5 months I had been walking in this new lifestyle of healthy eating and exercising. My scale said I had lost 4o pounds, and I had to buy clothing 2 sizes smaller than before. And these facts were validated by my friends and family, who also noticed the change. But there, standing in front of the mirror that day, I couldn't see what they saw. I still saw my body the same way as before: overweight and unattractive. What was going on? I knew I had lost weight because of the clothes and the numbers on the scale, yet my eyes saw no change from when I started. I should have been experiencing joy and celebrating; instead I was disappointed with the body image reflecting back at me. Why couldn't I see what others were seeing? I closed my eyes and prayed, "Lord, let me see the person you see." I wish I could tell you that when I opened my eyes I instantly saw the real physical me at that time, but instead God began slowly to reveal to me my heart.

You see, my heart was still clinging to what our culture deems to be an acceptable body image and weight. Our culture teaches us that if you are not that ideal you will not be accepted and you are not attractive. Because I was not fitting that mold, I didn't consider my body to be beautiful and acceptable. I still saw fat and not good enough.

> *But the* LORD *said to Samuel, "Do not consider his appearance or his height, for I have rejected him. The* LORD *does not look at the things people look at. People look at the outward appearance, but the* LORD *looks at the heart."*
>
> *1 Samuel 16:7 (NIV)*

Day 36 ~ Made in the Image of God

I was judging my body image and weight by the world's standards. My heart had adopted the lie that I needed to be a certain weight and look a certain way in order to be happy, satisfied, and accepted. The Lord knew it was my heart's belief in a lie that was influencing what I saw when I looked in the mirror. The eyes of my heart needed to be opened to the Truth before my physical eyes could be opened to see the real me.

So God created man in his own image, in the image of God he created him; male and female he created them.
                                                        Genesis 1:27 (NIV)

The Truth is that we are made in the likeness of God. We are not God, but we are made to be an image that reflects His beauty, peace, and love—a body created by Him and for Him (Colossians 1:16). God decided long before we were born exactly what we would look like (Psalm 139:13–16). And when God looks at what He has made, including us, He sees it as good. He is pleased with how He made *you* (Genesis 1:31). He designed our bodies with His purpose in mind, which is to bring Him glory in all we do.

So, when I stand in front of my mirror seeing my body as fat and not good enough, criticizing what I see and being dissatisfied, I am essentially telling God that His creation is not good enough and I am questioning whether God got it wrong. Imagine a piece of clay turning to the artist molding and shaping it into a pot saying, "Stop what you are doing; you messed me up with your clumsy hands." How absurd, right? That piece of clay was nothing until the artist envisioned its form and used his talented hands to create a beautiful vessel. God did the same with us: He envisioned our form, then created beautiful vessels: you and me. But we question and argue with God over his artistry in designing our image. And Isaiah warns us what will happen when we question what God has created.

What sorrow awaits those who argue with their Creator? Does a clay pot argue with its maker? Does the clay dispute with the one who shapes it, saying, "Stop, you're doing it wrong"? Does the pot exclaim, "How clumsy can you be?"
                                                        Isaiah 45:9 (NLT)

When we argue with, question, or doubt the goodness of God's creation, our bodies, we will find sorrow—a sorrow that brings disappointment and discontentment with our body image and weight; a sorrow that pulls us into a place where we are never satisfied with the gift God has given us: the gift of our bodies. And when we are not satisfied with our body image, we seek satisfaction in unhealthy ways, which leads to trashing the temple and stifling our souls.

In order to become satisfied with our body image and weight, we must first reject the world's definition of acceptable body image and weight, then allow the eyes of our hearts to be opened by the Truth that we are made in the image of God, an image of beauty, peace, and love, and that we were created for the purpose of reflecting His glory. Accepting that we are fearfully and wonderfully made leaves no room for arguing with our Creator about what He has created. But be careful: accepting your current body image and weight is not an excuse to neglect the temple, nor is it a reason to be prideful in our appearance. Striving to take care of our bodies by eating healthy, resting, and exercising is a worthy goal. It is one way we can demonstrate that we believe our image is valuable and acceptable. By making the goal of our weight loss and body image to reflect the glory of God, we can find confidence and contentment in our physical appearance regardless of the world's standards.

Taking It to Heart

1. What do you see when you look at yourself in the mirror?

Day 36 ~ Made in the Image of God

2. What cultural ideal of this world are you still clinging to that is influencing your body image and weight goals?

3. Does that ideal bring you satisfaction or disappointment when you look at yourself in the mirror?

4. How has your disappointment in your body image and weight manifested in unhealthy habits of eating, resting, and exercise?

5. What would it feel like to have confidence in and be content with your physical appearance?

6. What would you gain by having confidence and contentment?

7. How would having confidence and contentment change your weight loss and body image goals?

Heavenly Father and Daughter Time

Ask your Heavenly Father to begin to open the eyes of your heart so that you may see your true reflection when you look in the mirror.

Temple Tip of the Day

As you lose weight, either alter or donate the clothing that no longer fits you as an incentive to stay on track and move forward toward your goals. ≈

Day 37

Running Is Fun?

When I started my exercise program I began by taking prayer walks. Basically this is walking and praying at the same time, and I loved those prayer walks. I actually started to crave them. As I walked more, my pace gradually increased. My body was gaining strength and losing weight, which was enabling me to move a little quicker. Eventually my pace increased to the point where I was doing what is known as "speed walking." Then one day I thought to myself, this pace is almost as fast as running. So I figured, how hard could it be to run? So I ran. You know, I have heard stories of how when people run they feel this sense of accomplishment, strength, and freedom. Well, that was not me. When I ran for the first time all I could feel was labored breathing and sweat pouring from every part of my body, and all I sensed was a desire to get back home and collapse. So it is safe to say that my first experience with running was not as easy as I thought it would be. But it did not stop me from running again. I did it time after time, persevering through the physical challenges. The funny thing about perseverance is that the more you do it, the stronger you get. And that is what happened: my running pace increased to the point where now I can run with a sense of accomplishment, strength, and freedom.

Now I am not telling you that you need to run, but I am encouraging you to persevere. Because when we chose to persevere we are choosing to go through a time of suffering that has the potential to make us stronger, physically and spiritually.

> *We know that suffering produces perseverance; perseverance, character; and character, hope.*
>
> *Romans 5:3–4 (NIV)*

Faith and Fitness for Life

In this life we will have challenges and we can choose to allow God to use those challenges to build our character, deepen our trust in God, and give us hope for the future. Much like I did in my first attempt at running, we might feel exhausted by our challenges, but to persevere means to maintain a purpose in spite of difficulties. When I took that first run my purpose was to continue running until I got home. As Christians that is also our purpose: to continue to run the race, live out God's plan and purpose in our lives, persevere through the challenges, and hold on to our faith in Jesus Christ until we meet Him face to face.

I have fought the good fight. I have finished the race. I have kept the faith.
2 Timothy 4:7 (NIV)

At the end of my time on earth, these are the words I want to be able to say. How about you?

Taking It to Heart

1. Recall a time in your life when you demonstrated perseverance in the face of difficulties. What did you do to persevere?

Day 37 ~ Running Is Fun?

2. As you move forward past the 40 days of fasting, what challenges might you face with your eating and exercise?

3. How can your past experiences of persevering help you in the challenges you mentioned in response to question 2?

Heavenly Father and Daughter Time

Thank your Heavenly Father for the challenges that make you grow. Pray for strength in persevering as you run and finish the race to which God has called you.

Temple Tip for the Day

Challenge yourself in your exercise routine. Add 5 to 10 minutes to your cardio exercise and/or 10 to 30 stomach crunches and push-ups. ≈

Day 38

Feed Your Faith, Not Just Your Face

Have you ever noticed how simple it is to feed our faces every day and how much of a struggle it is to feed our faith every day? Eating comes so naturally, but prayer and reading the Word can often feel like a battle. Yet just like we need food to nourish our bodies and produce good health, we also need the Word of God to nourish our spirit and produce a healthy and prosperous soul.

> *All Scripture is God-breathed and is useful for teaching, rebuking, correcting and training in righteousness, so that the man of God may be thoroughly equipped for every good work.*
>
> *2 Timothy 3:16–17 (NIV)*

The Bible is our instruction manual for life. By reading it we come to know the Truth and understand the heart of God. It gives us guidance in making decisions and comfort in times of trouble. It is our source of knowing right from wrong and how to treat others. It is the nourishment we need for our spirit to grow and produce fruit.

I love to garden and right beside our deck is a small plot filled with some of my favorite perennial flowering plants. For years we have had a gorgeous Butterfly Bush that grows big and full of blooms in the summer. But last winter was hard on the plants and it appeared that the Butterfly Bush did not make it. For weeks we waited for signs of life, but all we saw were dry, brittle sticks where once there had been a green bush. We resigned ourselves to

Day 38 ~ Feed Your Faith

the fact that it was gone and decided that in the fall we would dig it out, because the root was so large and deep it would probably disturb the other plants if we took it out during the summer. Then one day we saw tiny little green shoots coming up from underneath the ground. At first I thought they were just weeds, but upon further inspection I realized it was the Butterfly Bush growing up again from its roots that were deep in the ground and had been protected from the harsh winter. I am happy to say the bush is now growing and thriving!

> *Let your roots grow down into him, and let your lives be built on him. Then your faith will grow strong in the truth you were taught, and you will overflow with thankfulness.*
>
> *Colossians 2:7 (NLT)*

When we feed our faith through prayer and studying the Word of God, our roots grow deep and large into Jesus and we are able to withstand the harsh moments of life. When we have a strong foundation built on God's Word we will grow strong in truth and be able to recognize and rebuke any lies the enemy may throw at us. Like the Butterfly Bush, when our faith roots are deep and large our spirits are well nourished and strong and will produce life—a healthy life.

> *Jesus answered by quoting Deuteronomy: "It takes more than bread to stay alive. It takes a steady stream of words from God's mouth."*
>
> *Matthew 4:4 (MSG)*

That is what we need to grow our roots deep and large: a steady stream of words from God's mouth into our hearts and minds, which means listening to His voice and meditating on His Word. Yes, we must take care of the Temple by being mindful of what we eat and how we exercise; but we also must be mindful daily to nourish our souls. This is God's desire for us: a healthy body and prosperous soul.

Taking It to Heart

1. How are you currently nourishing your soul?

2. What would it feel like to have your faith roots deep and large in Christ?

3. What step(s) could you take to grow your faith roots deep and large?

4. What might hinder you in taking those steps?

5. How can you minimize those hindrances?

Heavenly Father and Daughter Time

Ask your Heavenly Father to nourish your soul. Listen for His voice today. Pray your favorite scripture throughout the day.

Temple Tip for the Day

Avocados are high in fiber and healthy fats. They are a great alternative to meat at any meal. ≈

Day 39

Pass It On!

Wow! Can you believe there is only one more day left in this fast? How amazing God has been through this journey. I am sure if your journey was anything like mine you have much to be thankful for and might even be standing in awe of what God has done for you. No matter where you are on this journey, I know that God has given you a reason to brag about what He has done in your life. And I want to encourage you to brag away! Brag about God, that is!

That is what a testimony is for: to brag about God, to bring Him glory and draw people closer to Him. And He can do that through you and your testimony about this time of fasting and praying.

> *They overcame him by the blood of the Lamb and by the word of their testimony; they did not love their lives so much as to shrink from death.*
>
> *Revelation 12:11 (NIV)*

Our testimonies are meant to be shared because when we share them we overcome the enemy. Ultimately it was Jesus's sacrifice on the cross that defeated Satan once and for all, but each time we open our mouths and speak of God's glory in our life we promote the Good News of Jesus to more people. And that is how we overcome. Our testimonies can promote the Good News, but they can also bring comfort to others.

> *He comforts us in all our afflictions, so that we may be able to comfort those who are in any kind of affliction, through the comfort we*

ourselves receive from God. For as the sufferings of Christ overflow to us, so our comfort overflows through Christ.

2 Corinthians 1:4–5 (HCSB)

If there is one thing I have learned in the journey of faith and fitness it is that women everywhere have the same struggles. You and I are not the only ones who suffer from low self-esteem, weight problems, and food addictions. But when God comforts one of His girls in these areas, He wants His comfort to overflow from us to other women who need His help. I heard this question once and it has stuck with me: "Do you want to be a river or a reservoir?" Do you just want to hold on to and store up all that God has done for you? Or do you want it to flow through you to others? Hopefully your answer is you want to be a river, to overflow with God's workings in your life.

Now, some of you might be thinking, "I can't speak in front of people or write a book." That's OK. Don't try to put the delivery of your testimony in a box. There are just as many ways to share your testimony as there are stars in the sky, which are too numerous to count. There is no right or wrong way to share what God has done in your life.

"Pass It On"

*It only takes a spark to get a fire going,
and soon all those around can warm up in its glowing.
That's how it is with God's love
once you've experienced it;
you spread his love to everyone;
you want to pass it on.*[*]

We sang this song often in the church I grew up in, and I just love the lyrics. They sum up why we want to share our testimonies: because once we have experienced God's love and healing, we can't help but want to pass it on to others. Someone was

---

[*] By Kurt Kaiser. © 1969 Communiqué Music, Inc. All rights reserved.

Faith and Fitness for Life

once the spark that ignited the fire in you; go be a spark and ignite others to practice faith and fitness for the Lord!

Taking It to Heart

1. Take time to look back and notice all that God has done for you during this time of fasting.

Day 39 ~ Pass It On!

2. Begin to write your testimony about your journey. Write about where you were when you started, what your goal was, how God provided for you during this time, what your challenges were, and how God delivered you from those challenges. Brag about God!

Heavenly Father and Daughter Time

Pray and ask your Heavenly Father for opportunities to begin sharing your testimony. Allow Him to show you how to share and with whom to share it.

Temple Tip for the Day

Junk food cravings can sneak up on you when you're feeling tired. Take a nap instead of grabbing for the junk food. ≈

Day 40

Time to Celebrate!!!

May he grant your heart's desires and make all your plans succeed. May we shout for joy when we hear of your victory and raise a victory banner in the name of our God. May the LORD answer all your prayers.

Psalm 20:4–5 (NLT)

Congratulations! You did it: 40 days of fasting and prayer and fitness. I am shouting for joy and raising a victory banner in the name of Jesus for all that He has done in and through you! You have been successful in fasting from the white stuff, exercising, and praying for 40 days, and I pray that your heart's desires have been granted. I know that strongholds have been broken and faith has been built, and I praise the Lord for these mighty works that He has done in you.

Perhaps many of you are wondering: now what? And that's a good question. What happens next depends on what God is asking you to do to maintain your healthy temple.

You're blessed when you stay on course, walking steadily on the road revealed by God. You're blessed when you follow his directions, doing your best to find him.

Psalm 119:1–2 (MSG)

Only God can answer the question, "Now what?" It is up to you to listen and walk in obedience the course He lays in front of you. I believe you can do all that God is asking of you through the power and strength of Jesus Christ.

Day 40 ~ Time to Celebrate!!!

It has been my privilege to be a part of your journey and I would love to hear about your challenges and successes. Your journey is not over because we hit day 40; in fact, it has only begun. So I would like to pray this for you:

> I pray that you continue to walk in His ways and desire to do what is pleasing to Him. I pray that you do your best and let God do the rest. I pray that you find a renewed motivation in taking care of God's temple, your body. I pray that you live out your identity as a daughter of the King. I pray that you allow God to be in your places of hurt and that you let His healing take place, and that you allow Him to share in the victories as well, giving Him all the glory and honor. I pray that you allow God to use you and your gifts, talents, and abilities to be a blessing to others. I pray that you may have good health and a prosperous soul. And finally:
>
> > *Now to him who is able to do immeasurably more than all we ask or imagine, according to his power that is at work within us, to him be glory in the church and in Christ Jesus throughout all generations, for ever and ever! Amen.*
> >
> > *Ephesians 3:20 (NIV)*

Taking It to Heart

1. Where you successful in meeting your goal(s) that you set on Day 1?

2. Why or why not?

3. What part(s) of the fast did you find most beneficial?

4. What part(s) of the fast did not help you at all?

5. What roadblocks did you encounter?

Day 40 ~ Time to Celebrate!!!

6. How might the benefits help you decide how to move forward?

Heavenly Father and Daughter Time

Spend time consulting your Heavenly Father on how He would like you to continue. Ask Him for specifics concerning your eating, exercise, and faith development.

Temple Tip for the Day

Take time to celebrate what God has achieved in and through you in these 40 days. Be creative, and have fun!!! ≈

Glossary of Bible Translations

AMP ≈ Amplified Bible
CEV ≈ Contemporary English Version
ESV ≈ English Standard Version
HCSB ≈ Holman Christian Standard Bible
KJV ≈ King James Version
MSG ≈ The Message
NASB ≈ New American Standard Bible
NIV ≈ New International Version
NLT ≈ New Living Translation
TLB ≈ The Living Bible

Also produced by
Not Forgotten Publishing Services

Born Again in Medjugorje: A Memoir
by Mary Hendel McCafferty, June 2012

The Quarry: A Novel
by Robert Carson, July 2012

Nan & Clete . . . and Then There Was One:
Finding a New Normal After a Traumatic Death
by Nancy S. Gibble, February 2013

Forget Me Not: A Tough and Tender Memoir
by Loraine Seavey Nixon Martin, March 2013

In God's Mercy: My Spiritual Journey
by Linda Lint, May 2013

The Little Society of St. Rita Prayer Book
by The Little Society of St. Rita, July 2013

The Notebooks of the Reverend
Damien Marie Saintourens, OP
by the Cloistered Dominican Nuns of the Perpetual Rosary,
Lancaster, PA, October 2013

Help the Homeless OFF THE STREETS
One Person at a Time
by Deacon Michael J. Oles, June 2014

Begin by Loving Again: My Safari
from Farm Girl to Missionary Doctor to Wife and Mother
by Dorcas L. Stoltzfus Morrow, M.D., September 2015

Not.Forgotten.Publishing@gmail.com

Made in the USA
Charleston, SC
23 September 2015